GASTROINTESTINAL BLEEDING
Diagnosis and Management

CLINICAL GASTROENTEROLOGY MONOGRAPH SERIES

John M. Dietschy, M.D., *Series Editor*

Gastrointestinal Bleeding: Diagnosis and Management
John A. Balint, M.B., F.R.C.P.
I. James Sarfeh, M.D.
Martin B. Fried, M.D.

Diseases of the Gallbladder and Biliary System
Leslie J. Schoenfield, M.D.

Complications of Gastric Surgery
David Fromm, M.D.

GASTROINTESTINAL BLEEDING
Diagnosis and Management

JOHN A. BALINT, M.B., F.R.C.P.
I. JAMES SARFEH, M.D.
MARTIN B. FRIED, M.D.

Albany Medical College
Albany, New York

A Wiley Medical Publication
John Wiley & Sons
New York ● London ● Sydney ● Toronto

Library of Congress Cataloging in Publication Data:

Balint, John A
  Gastrointestinal bleeding.

  (Clinical gastroenterology monograph series) (A Wiley medical publication)
  Includes bibliographical references and index.
  1. Gastrointestinal hemorrhage. I. Sarfeh, I. James, joint author. II. Fried, Martin Barry, 1946- joint author. III. Title. IV. Series. [DNLM: 1. Hemorrhage, Gastrointestinal—Diagnosis. 2. Hemorrhage, Gastrointestinal—Therapy. WI143 B186g]

  RC802.B34   616.3'3   77-4423
  ISBN 0-471-04607-8

Printed in the United States of America

10 9 8 7 6 5 4 3 2 1

to
Sir Francis Avery Jones, M.D., F.R.C.P.
Physician, Teacher, Investigator, and Friend

SERIES PREFACE

During the past decade remarkable progress has been made in our understanding of many basic physiological processes related to liver and gastrointestinal tract functions. Much of this information has led to significant improvements in our understanding of clinical diseases that alter normal hepatic and intestinal function and in the therapy of these diseases. Innumerable examples can be cited. For instance, the application of basic principles of physical chemistry has clarified considerably the manner in which cholesterol is solubilized in bile. Related studies have identified the causes of cholesterol gallstones in several large groups of patients, and specific forms of therapy for the prevention or the dissolution of such stones are now available. Other experimental work that relies heavily on basic techniques of immunology and electron microscopy has identified specific infectious agents affecting liver function. These studies, in turn, have provided considerable insight into the different clinical syndromes included under the general heading of viral hepatitis, raising the possibility that effective immunization against these organisms may soon be available. Equally impressive advances have been made in our understanding of the control of gastric secretion and peptic ulcer disease, in the causes of intestinal malabsorption, and in radiographic and endoscopic methods for examining the liver and gastrointestinal tract.

This explosion of knowledge in gastroenterology poses a particularly difficult problem for those interested in the dissemination of new medical information to students, house officers and medical practitioners. Often advances have come so quickly that the information presented in standard textbooks is outdated before the books become available. Also, it is difficult to revise such texts rapidly because of the large number of authors involved and the long production time necessary for these books. Finally, the space available to authors for extensively reviewing both the basic physiological concepts and their clinical implications is limited in most texts and in more rapidly published medical journals.

This series of volumes published under the general title "Clinical Gastroenterology Monographs" was conceived and designed to overcome many of these difficulties and to bring to the medical practitioner the most current information on the pathophysiology and treatment of major areas of disease affecting the liver and gastrointestinal tract. Each volume covers an important group of related disorders and is sufficiently long to allow for extensive discussion of their basic pathophysiological, clinical, and therapeutic aspects. New volumes will appear regularly, and a special effort will be made to identify areas for inclusion in the series in which there is a rapidly expanding body of information relevant to the care of patients with a particular gastrointestinal disorder. Existing volumes will be updated and republished frequently where continued advances in information justify such rapid revision.

It is hoped that this series will provide a continuously evolving and current reference source for the broad spectrum of physicians who deal with patients with diseases of the liver and gastrointestinal tract.

John M. Dietschy, M.D.

PREFACE

The patient presenting with gastrointestinal hemorrhage poses a difficult diagnostic and management problem for the physician. During the past 15 years major advances have been made in these fields. The developments in both fiberoptic endoscopy and selective angiography have provided the physician with the means to make a precise and specific diagnosis as to the origin of bleeding. A greater understanding of the physiologic and biochemical consequences of acute hemorrhage has created a basis for better management of patients with major hemorrhage. New surgical approaches have also been developed. These diagnostic and treatment modalities and pathophysiological insights have now been available long enough to permit an assessment of their contribution. On the basis of such an evaluation, we offer a logical and practical approach to the problem.

A problem-oriented format is utilized. We indicate where decisions are based on hard data and where they are made on the basis of clinical impressions. Where appropriate, we review the physiological and biochemical changes that are important to an understanding of the clinical disorder or its management.

Our aim is to present important basic concepts with particular emphasis on the more common and major diseases. We do not attempt to be all-inclusive; readers should refer to specific texts for detailed descriptions of disease entities. Finally, and perhaps most importantly, the book presents the views of an internist, gastroenterologist, and surgeon, a team that we believe is crucial for the optimal care of patients with gastrointestinal bleeding.

JOHN A. BALINT, M.D.

Albany, New York
March, 1977

ACKNOWLEDGMENTS

I have had help from many friends in the writing of this book. My thanks are due especially to my wife, who patiently proofread and edited the manuscript; to Mrs. Marcia Novak, who cheerfully and efficiently retyped it many times; and to Sir Francis Avery Jones, who enthusiastically supplied me with important references. Without their invaluable assistance this volume would have taken much, much longer to prepare.

JOHN A. BALINT

CONTENTS

GASTROINTESTINAL BLEEDING
Diagnosis and Management

1
GENERAL CONSIDERATIONS

The proper management of the patient with gastrointestinal bleeding involves a series of important decisions, each based on the accurate clinical assessment of the problem at hand. Many of these steps are based on sound physiologic or epidemiologic principles. Others, however, are based more on art, or, if you will, dogma, than on hard scientific fact. Thus the management of the patient presenting with bleeding from the gastrointestinal tract involves both the science and the art of medicine. Our purpose in this book is to present our view of the principles that should guide the physician in caring for such a patient. We indicate where these principles are based on hard data and also where they are derived from clinical impressions. Whenever possible, we present the approach to patients with gastrointestinal bleeding in a problem-solving format and, when appropriate, indicate alternative positions that have been recommended.

The year 1935 marked a major turning point in the management of patients with gastrointestinal hemorrhage. In that year two reports appeared that laid the foundations for our present mode of treatment of these patients. Meulengracht (1) reported on his experience with 251 patients treated with a regimen of pureed diet, antacids, sedation, and oral iron replacement starting within 24 hours of admission to the hospital. There were only three deaths (1.5%). By contrast in a comparable group of 289 patients treated in a neighboring Copenhagen hospital with the old regime of ice chips only, the mortality was 7.9%. Most other investigators at that time using the old regime reported mortality rates of 11 to 25% (1). Meulengracht listed his reasons for trying diet therapy as follows:

1. Exhausted patients were likely to die.
2. Bleeding sometimes seemed to stop with feeding.
3. Ambulant patients with melena often stopped bleeding on their own.
4. It seemed to him unreasonable to starve patients who needed food *and* fluids.

This requirement for fluid and blood replacement presented a major problem until in the same year Marriott and Kekwick (2) reported on a method for the continuous drip infusion of blood. Intravenous infusion of electrolyte solutions had first been used 100 years earlier by Drs. O'Shaughnessy and Latta to treat the dehydration of cholera, but it had fallen into disrepute because of problems with infections. Blood transfusions had been used early in this century when blood grouping was first established in 1901 by Landsteiner so that this form of therapy could be safely undertaken. However, until 1935 blood transfusions involved direct intravenous injection of freshly drawn blood. This limited the usefulness of transfusion. Marriott and Kekwick (2) described a method for controlled, prolonged infusion of large amounts of blood by a method that in its essentials is still in use today. They described their experience with 17 patients given between 2.6 and 6.6 liters of blood. Their description of the change in their first patient is impressive testimony to the benefits of this new treatment modality. "His demeanor changed from that of a dying man to an optimistic invalid." The patient had ulcerative colitis.

As illustrated by this case, gastrointestinal bleeding is always a potentially life threatening condition. When the patient presents with a massive hemorrhage and shows evidence of circulatory embarrassment, this threat is evident. However, even a relatively small bleeding episode may presage a later massive hemorrhage. Alternatively, even mild or occult bleeding, which is not in itself a threat to the patient's life, may be the presenting symptom or sign of a major illness, such as gastric carcinoma. Yet, again, a bleeding episode may complicate a relatively benign condition, such as acute peptic ulcer. Each of these general situations requires different approaches to therapy. Therefore, appropriate management decisions will depend on precise diagnosis as to the site and pathologic nature of the bleeding lesion, the magnitude of the hemorrhage, and the presence or absence of complicating conditions. Thus the problem is predictably greater in older patients than in younger individuals. It is only when all the necessary facts are assembled and carefully reviewed, that correct decisions about treatment can be made. Since gathering the necessary data will usually involve the internist, the endoscopist (gastroenterologist), and the radiologist, although treatment may well be surgical, a team approach is basic to good management, and it should be instituted at the earliest possible time.

DEFINITIONS

Gastrointestinal hemorrhage may be massive, overt, or occult, and may come from any part of the digestive tract. *Massive bleeding* may be defined quantitatively or functionally. The presence of signs of circulatory embarrassment indicates massive blood loss. These signs include hypotension, tachycardia, peripheral vasoconstriction, and oliguria. Alternatively, a patient requiring 2500 ml or more of blood replacement in the first 24 hours is considered as having had a massive hemorrhage. *Overt bleeding* is defined as the occurrence of hematemesis (i.e., the vomiting of blood), melena (i.e., the passage of black, tarry stools), or of bright red rectal bleeding, not requiring massive blood replacement, and not associated with signs of circulatory embarrassment. The presence of positive tests for occult blood in the stools with or without associated anemia is evidence of *occult gastrointestinal bleeding.*

SITE OF BLEEDING

Hemorrhage may originate from any part of the digestive tract. As a first step in diagnosis, it is helpful to determine from which general area of the gastrointestinal tract the bleeding is coming. Thus the upper gastrointestinal tract is taken to include the esophagus, stomach, and duodenum. *Upper gastrointestinal bleeding* usually presents with melena with or without hematemesis which may be massive. Bleeding from the upper digestive tract is often associated with symptoms of the causative lesion such as peptic ulcer, cirrhosis of the liver or esophagitis. *Lower gastrointestinal bleeding* usually presents with passage of red blood per rectum, since it originates in the large bowel. Such bleeding is rarely massive and may be otherwise asymptomatic, unless it is due to inflammatory bowel disease. *Bleeding from the small bowel* is uncommon compared with hemorrhage from the upper or lower gastrointestinal tract. The bleeding is rarely massive and is often occult. It is often unassociated with symptoms other than those due to blood loss.

ETIOLOGIC CONSIDERATIONS

Within each of these three areas of the gastrointestinal tract certain lesions are common causes of overt bleeding, but others rarely result in such events. Thus, acute superficial mucosal lesions are responsible for about 25% of upper gastrointestinal bleeds (3,4), while carcinoma of the stomach accounts for only about 2% (5). Armed with this type of data, examination can be directed specifically to elicit information relative to the likely cause of bleeding. This information is important not only in providing the basis for therapeutic decisions but also in indicating the special investigative procedures most likely to help in establishing the diagnosis. Furthermore, the preliminary diagnosis provides information on which to base the prognosis and the proper management.

MAJOR DECISIONS

The most important decision in any patient with gastrointestinal bleeding is whether treatment is to be medical or surgical. The importance of this decision is well illustrated by the results reported by Gordon-Taylor in the first Lettsomian Lecture to the Medical Society of London in 1946 (6). Even in those early days of the surgical treatment of bleeding peptic ulcer, he was asked to see about 20% of such patients during their admission. He reported that he was able to operate successfully, with a 5.5% mortality, if he was asked to see the patient early. When he was asked to see the patient late, and to operate as a desperate measure to save the patient's life, the mortality rate rose to 36%. The timing of the decision on whether a patient is to be treated medically or surgically is thus very important. This decision will depend on the answers to several questions:

1. Is the lesion causing bleeding amenable to surgical management?

2. Is the patient an acceptable surgical risk? The patient's age, clinical condition, and the presence of complicating associated diseases are major determinants of the answer to this question.

3. What is the magnitude of the blood loss? Estimates of volume depletion depend on clinical judgement, supplemented when necessary by special investigation such as measurements of central venous pressure.

4. Does the patient require intensive resuscitative measures? Stabilization of the patient's circulatory status is a prerequisite to establishing a precise diagnosis and to all other therapeutic undertakings.

The answers to these questions and the decisions based on them require a team approach by the internist, endoscopist, radiologist, and surgeon. The role of these members of the team have been significantly altered in recent years. The internist has been provided with the means to provide adequate fluid and blood replacement, and the surgeon has at his disposal a variety of surgical procedures developed during the past 20 years. The role of the endoscopist was dramatically changed by the advent of the fiberoptic instruments (7). In 1952 Avery Jones (8) felt that gastroscopy was no substitute for radiologic examination. However, that statement was based on experience with the semirigid instruments then available. The new fiberoptic instruments together with newer analgesic drugs, such as Diazepam, make for greater patient comfort and much better visualization of the esophagus, stomach, and duodenum in a single evaluation. Thus, endoscopy now offers complete evaluation of the upper gastrointestinal tract with the ability to make precise diagnoses (9). Radiologists have also been provided with a new diagnositc and, indeed, therapeutic, method by the advent of selective abdominal angiography (10). This procedure provides not only a method for localizing the site of bleeding but also a means for its control in selected instances. Thus we now have the means of making precise diagnoses and of controlling hemorrhage. As a result we gain time for the resuscitation of the patient before undertaking definitive surgical treatment of the problem if this is indicated.

REFERENCES

1. Meulengracht, E.: Treatment of hematemesis and melena with food. *Lancet,* **2:**1220, 1935.
2. Marriott, H. L. and A. Kekwick: Continuous drip blood transfusion. *Lancet,* **1:**977, 1935.
3. Palmer, E. D.: The vigorous diagnostic approach to upper gastrointestinal tract hemorrhage. A 23 year prospective study of 1400 cases. *JAMA,* **207:**1477, 1969.
4. Gordon, H. E. Moderator UCLA, Interdepartmental Conference: Diagnosis and management of gastrointestinal bleeding. *Ann. Intern. Med.* **71:**993, 1969.
5. Schiller, K. F. R., Truelove, S. C., and G. D. Williams: Hematemesis and melena with special reference to factors influencing outcome. *Brit. Med. J.* **2:**7, 1970.
6. Gordon-Taylor, G.: Present position of surgery in the treatment of bleeding peptic ulcer. *Brit. J. Surg.* **33:**336, 1946.
7. Hirschowitz, B. I.: Endoscopic examination of the stomach and duodenal cap with the fiberscope. *Lancet* **1:**1074, 1961.
8. Jones, F. A.: *Modern Trends in Gastroenterology.* Butterworth and Co., Ltd., London, 1952.
9. Colcher, H.: Guidelines for fiberoptic examination in upper gastro-intestinal bleeding. *Adv. Intn. Med.* **20:**399, 1975.
10. Baum, S, Athanasoulis, C. A., Waltman, A. C., and E. J. Rug: Gastrointestinal hemorrhage, II. Angiographic diagnosis and control. *Adv. Surgery,* **7:**149, 1973.

2

PRESENTATION AND CLINICAL DIAGNOSIS

In this chapter, we deal with the four major presentations in gastrointestinal bleeding (i.e., hematemesis, melena, red rectal bleeding, and occult bleeding) separately. Although the approaches to the patient with each of these presentations will overlap, there are differences that warrant separate discussion of each.

UPPER GASTROINTESTINAL BLEEDING

Jean Cruveilhier in his "Anatomie Pathologique du corps Humaine" (Paris, 1830–42) first fully described peptic ulcer and presented a classic description of a young man who died of hemorrhage from a gastric ulcer in the antrum (1). The patient was a muscular young carpenter of 29 years with a long history of alcoholic excess. Five years earlier he had bled repeatedly but recovered. He then did well in the interval, although he returned to drinking. On April 15, 1830, burning epigastric pain developed. On the 30th he began to vomit blood and was admitted to the Charite. Here he was found to be in shock (small pulse, easily compressed and severe anemia) so that he could not be bled! Next day he was a little better, but on May 2 he had a massive further hematemesis and died. At autopsy a large, chronic ulcer was found with an artery in its base. This case history is indeed a classical presentation, and it illustrates many of the problems in clinical diagnosis and decision making that face the physician when he first sees a patient with hematemesis.

Hematemesis (Scheme 2-1)

In this patient the problem was presented as overt bleeding evidenced by hematemesis. As shown in Scheme 2-1, this presentation allows the conclusion that bleeding has occurred from the upper gastrointestinal tract, that is, from a point above the ligament of Treitz. While it is true that bleeding from this area of the gastrointestinal tract may not result in hematemesis, bleeding beyond the ligament of Treitz rarely will result in vomiting of blood. Cruveilhier's patient had a history of excessive alcohol intake, but also complained of burning epigastric pain. Thus, on historical grounds a diagnosis of esophageal varices, gastritis, or of peptic ulcer must be considered. However, more importantly, examination showed the patient to be in an unstable circulatory state. This finding mandates immediate steps to correct

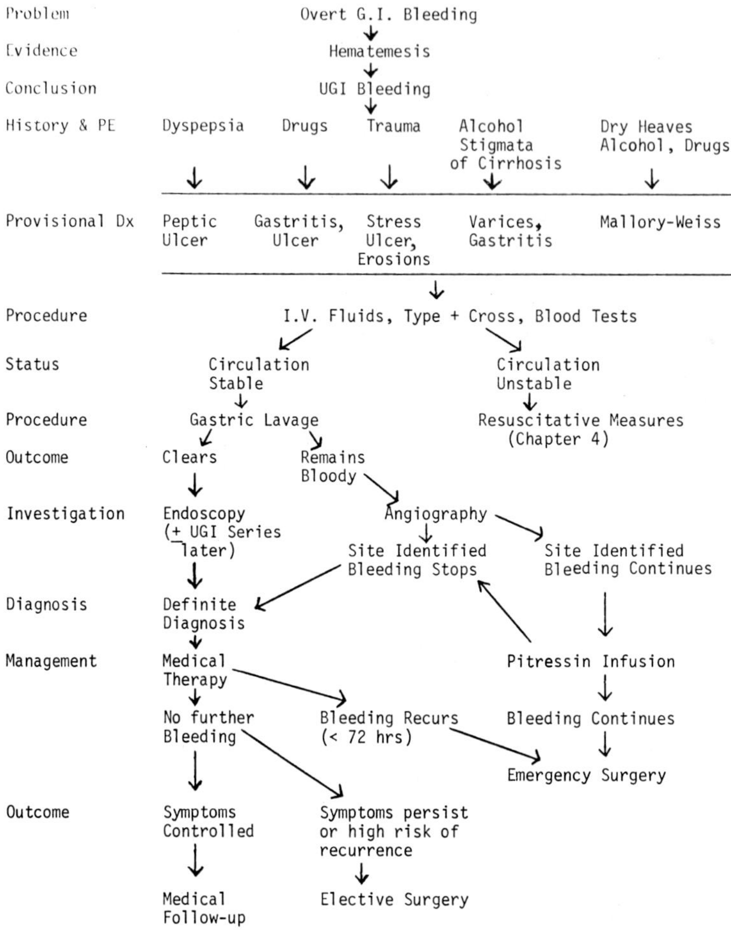

SCHEME 2-1

the volume deficit before further diagnostic evaluation is undertaken. The evaluation of circulatory status and the considerations involved in correction of this situation are discussed in Chapter 4.

Provisional clinical diagnosis

If the patient's circulatory status is stable, a full history and physical examination is undertaken. The history should include careful inquiry for symptoms suggesting peptic ulcer, previous gastric surgery, drug ingestion, alcoholic excess, recent trauma or infection, retching, blood disorders, and family history. The relative frequency of major causative lesions will vary somewhat from country to country. Table 2-1 has been constructed from data presented by Palmer based on his prospective study of 1400 patients over 23 years in the United States (2) and by Schiller, Truelove, and Williams from a study of 2149 patients studied in Oxford, England (3). In both series, duodenal ulcer was thought to be the source of bleeding in about 30% of the patients. Gastric ulcer was the bleeding site in 12% to 15% of

Table 2-1
Major Causes of Upper Gastrointestinal Bleeding

Disease	Cardinal Features	Age	Frequency (%)	
			(2)*	(3)*
Duodenal ulcer Gastric ulcer	Periodic bouts of pain Relief from food or antacids Relief of pain with bleeding	> 20	27.7 12.6	29.0 15.1
Gastritis	Salicylates, steroids, alcohol, dyspepsia	Any age	12.0	—
Esophageal varices	Alcohol, previous liver disease, hepatomegaly, stigmata of cirrhosis	Any age	18.7	2.4
Mallory-Weiss	Dyspepsia, dry heaves, alcohol	Any age	5.7	—
Carcinoma of stomach	Anorexia, weight loss	> 40	—	2.2
Other			23.3	51.3†

*Based on data from references 2 and 3.
†Includes 26.2% undiagnosed sources of bleeding.

instances. Esophageal varices, secondary to hepatic cirrhosis, were diagnosed as causing bleeding in 18.7% of Palmer's patients (2), but only in 2.4% of the British series (3). This difference presumably reflects the different prevalence of alcoholic liver disease in the two countries. Mallory-Weiss syndrome (4), that is, esophageal mucosal tears, was reported to be the cause of bleeding in 5.7% of patients by Palmer (2), who used esophagogastroscopy regularly. This lesion was not noted by Schiller et al. (3) who did not use endoscopy frequently. Others have reported esophageal tears in some 10% of patients with upper gastrointestinal bleeding (5). It is important to note that carcinoma of the stomach, esophagus, or duodenum was found to account for only about 2% of bleeding episodes (2,3). The converse of this is also true, in that only about 2% of gastric carcinomas bleed overtly. Thus malignant lesions of the stomach are rare causes of major, overt bleeding. As we discuss later, such lesions commonly give rise to occult bleeding. Hence the major causes of hemorrhage listed in Table 2-1 account for about 80% of all cases. Another lesion that is being recognized with increasing frequency is the so-called stress ulcer (6,7,8,9). This lesion occurs in the stomach, and also in the duodenum. It develops in patients who have suffered massive trauma, cerebral injury, severe burns, or major infections and is a dreaded complication in these situations. It is most commonly encountered in hospitalized patients, with bleeding occurring 4 to 15 days after admission.

Peptic ulcer.   Overt hemorrhage is a common complication of peptic ulcer, with an incidence of about 1% per annum, as reported in most series (10,11). Peptic ulcer has its peak prevalence rate in the fourth and fifth decade of life. Bleeding from this cause may be suspected on clinical grounds in a majority of instances. The patient often has a very helpful history of periodic indigestion and antacid ingestion. Typically, the dyspeptic symptoms, especially pain, increase for several days before the onset of bleeding and promptly subside once hemorrhage has occurred. Some-times, these events follow a period of stress. The bleeding episode may present as hematemesis, melena, or both.

There are no specific physical findings of peptic ulcer other than epigastric tenderness and rarely a distended stomach. Physical examination is important, how-ever, in confirming the absence of physical findings of other causes of bleeding or of associated disease. Finally, the history and physical examination are most important in determining the circulatory status of the patient, as is described in the discussion that follows.

Gastritis.   This diagnosis should be suspected in patients who present with upper gastrointestinal bleeding following recent heavy ingestion of alcoholic bever-ages, salicylates, or perhaps adrenocorticosteroid medication, and may affect pa-tients of all ages. The association of gastritis with alcohol abuse is well recognized. It is, however, difficult to differentiate this lesion as a cause of bleeding from that caused by esophageal varices on clinical grounds alone, and endoscopic confirmation will be needed. The association of salicylate ingestion with gastritis and, indeed, peptic ulcer and hemorrhage has become accepted in recent years (12,13). Since salicylates appear in many over-the-counter medications, inquiry for their use has to be rather searching, or the patient may well not recognize that a medication contains salicylates. As in the case of ulcer disease, the physical examina-tion is crucial in evaluating the circulatory state of the patient and excluding other causes of bleeding.

Esophageal varices.   Hemorrhage from esophageal varices may vary from mas-sive to mild and recurrent. There is usally a history of alcohol abuse or previous liver disease. In children, with the possibility of extrahepatic portal obstruction, the ques-tion of umbilical infection should be investigated. Physical examination should be directed to finding evidence of portal hypertension such as splenomegaly, dilated abdominal wall veins, and ascites. The liver is often enlarged, and there may be spider angiomata on the skin. Since, however, the spleen will contract in response to hemorrhage, splenomegaly may not be appreciated. In addition, the patient is often jaundiced. The physical findings in patients with esophageal bleeding not only help to suggest the diagnosis but also indicate whether the patient is an acceptable candi-date for surgical therapy. Thus, the presence of marked jaundice, ascites, bruising, and evidence of hepatic encephalopathy make the patient a poor surgical risk.

Mallory-Weiss syndrome.   This condition, which may occur at any age, classically presents with a history of repeated retching or dry heaves followed by hematemesis (4). Alcohol abuse is a frequent precipitating factor. However, other causes of gastritis may also lead to esophageal mucosal tears. Usually there is no clear history of previous dyspepsia. Physical findings are unremarkable, other than those at-tributable to the hemorrhage.

Carcinoma of the stomach.   This condition, as indicated in Table 2 .1, is a rare cause of massive gastrointestinal bleeding. However, ulcerating carcinomas may lead to major bleeding episodes. The patient is usually over 50 years of age, with a short history of dyspepsia that is often accompanied by anorexia and striking weight loss. It should be remembered that giant ulcers (greater than 2.5 cm in diameter) are more often benign than malignant. Final diagnosis needs confirmation by endoscopy and by four-quadrant biopsy of the edges of the ulcer after hemorrhage has been arrested for several days.

Other causes of upper gastrointestinal bleeding.   These are presented in Table 2-2. The so-called *stress ulcers* first described as an entity by Curling in 1842 are perhaps the most common in this category (6-9). These lesions develop in 2% to 3% of patients with massive trauma, sepsis, burns, or cerebral lesions (6-9). Most often bleeding from these ulcers, which are commonly multiple, occurs 2 to 15 days after hospitalization. This is a particularly grave situation, since it occurs in an already seriously ill patient. Beil et al (7) in 1962 reported an overall mortality of 71% in their 35 subjects. The outlook in this group of patients has been improved by the availability of intraarterial pitressin infusion.

Leaking aneurysms or from infected aortic grafts and mesenteric vascular occlusions.   These are fortunately rare causes of gastrointestinal hemorrhage and tend to occur in older patients with vascular disease. Prompt diagnosis, however, gives the only hope of saving the patient's life. The diagnosis is often very difficult. A high index of suspicion is needed, especially in patients with evidence of arteriosclerotic cardiovascular disease, or cardiac arrhythmia. If there is a history of severe postprandial abdominal pain and weight loss preceding the bleeding episode, the level of suspicion should be even higher. The presence of abdominal or femoral arterial bruits, and a pulsatile mass in the abdomen are highly suggestive physical findings for aneurysm. Gastrointestinal bleeding in the face of a silent abdomen is very suggestive of mesenteric vascular occlusion, especially if a perforation can be ruled out.

Osler-Weber-Rendu syndrome (telengiectasia).   This usually presents with a history of repeated bleeding, often occult, in a patient with no history of other sources of bleeding. The diagnosis can usually be established by careful examination of the mucous membranes for the telltale vascular lesions. It is important to examine the patient for these lesions after restoration of blood volume, since the telengiectases may not be apparent when the patient is first seen.

The other lesions listed with their cardinal features in Table 2-2 are even rarer. Many of these lesions can be readily recognized on careful examination of the patient as indicated. Some of them will be discussed further in relation to obscure gastrointestinal bleeding in Chapter 6.

Investigation

After a preliminary clinical diagnosis has been arrived at, a decision must be taken whether the patient is in a stable or unstable circulatory state. In the latter case, the patient will be treated as discussed in Chapter 4. If, however, the patient's status is stable, that is skin turgor is good, pulse pressure is 30 mm Hg or greater, diastolic pressure is >60 mm Hg and pulse rate not excessive, further investigation to ascertain the source of bleeding may be pursued. Before this is undertaken, an intravenous infusion of isotonic electrolyte solution should be started. At the same

Table 2-2
Less Common Causes of Upper Gastrointestinal Bleeding

Disease	*Cardinal Features*	*Age*
A. Diseases amenable to surgical treatment		
Stress ulcers and erosive gastritis	Follow 2 to 15 days after severe burns, surgery, trauma or brain injury, sepsis	Any age
Aortic aneurysm	Massive bleeding, but may have recurrent episodes	> 40
A-V malformations	Isolated episodes of x-ray negative hemorrhage	Any age
Mesenteric vascular occlusion	Acute abdominal catastrophy, bleeding with silent abdomen	> 40
Hemobilia	Biliary colic, jaundice, bleeding	Any age
Benign and malignant tumors of small bowel	Often have painless, recurrent bleeding May have cramping pain	Any age
B. Diseases requiring medical management		
Heredofamilial		
Osler-Weber-Rendu (Telengiectasia)	Often familial, history of nose bleeds recurrent bleeding; telengiectasia	Any age
Pseudoxanthoma elasticum	Tigroid (angioid) streaking of retina, Morocco leather skin, BP ↑	< 50
Ehlers-Danlos	Abnormal skin elasticity Hyperextensible joints	< 50
Hematologic diseases		
Hemophilia	History of bleeding disorder	
Von Willebrand's disease	Cutaneous or joint hemorrhages	Any age
Thrombocytopenia*	Purpura, splenomegaly	
Lymphoma*	Hematologic abnormalities, splenomegaly	
Disseminated intravascular coagulation	Often have liver disease or severe infection	Any age
Fibrinolysis	Abnormal clotting tests	
Drugs		
Anticoagulants	Absence of other causes,	Any age
Reserpine	history of drug ingestion	
Salicylates	abnormal clotting tests	

*Some forms of thrombocytopenia, and lymphomas if localized, may be amenable to surgical treatment.

time, blood should be obtained for typing and crossmatching. Other items for the data base should include serum electrolytes, prothrombin time, activated partial thromboplastin time, blood urea nitrogen, hemoglobin, hematocrit, and platelet count. An electrocardiogram and chest radiograph should also be obtained. The patient's urine output must be monitored and intravenous fluid replacement rate adjusted to maintain a urine output of 50 ml per hr or greater. At the same time the patient's cardiac status should be watched especially in those over 50 years of age, or with evidence of heart disease, so as to avoid fluid overload.

While these steps are being initiated, consultation should be obtained with a gastroenterologist or endoscopist and a surgeon. It is most important that further decisions about the management of the patient should be made in concert by all those whose services may be needed in the treatment of this individual. It is also advisable to consider alerting the radiologist about the presence of the patient, so as to avoid undue delay should angiography or barium contrast studies become necessary on an urgent basis.

As indicated in Scheme 2-1, a nasogastric or orogastric tube should then be passed. It is best to use a large (F16) Salem sump or Ewald tube. This permits the gastric content to be aspirated. The presence of gross blood in the gastric aspirate, whether fresh or altered (coffee grounds) confirms the presence of upper gastrointestinal hemorrhage. The stomach is then lavaged with saline. Many authorities recommend the use of iced saline, since it is thought that the cooling effect will reduce mucosal blood flow and thus help arrest bleeding. There are, however, no good data to substantiate this claim. We believe that such lavage is valuable mainly in emptying the stomach of blood clot, thus allowing it to contract. If lavage is successful in emptying the stomach of blood so that the returns become clear, further investigation by means of upper gastrointestinal panendoscopy becomes possible. If the returns remain bloody, this procedure will not be feasible and a decision as to angiography will have to be taken. This topic is discussed in Chapter 3.

The value of early panendoscopy is still a subject of debate. According to Schiller et al (3), 78.6% of patients with peptic ulcer bleed only once during a particular hospital admission for hemorrhage. These patients could, therefore, be handled very conservatively without seriously impairing their chance of full recovery. However, it is not easy to predict which patient will fall into this group when first seen. Avery Jones (14,15) suggested that the risk of recurrent bleeding may be increased in patients over 50 years of age with chronic peptic ulcers and ulcer pain that persists after the onset of bleeding. These observations are supported in part by the data of Lewin and Truelove (16), which showed a steeply rising mortality with increasing age. However, these authors found no evidence to support the idea that the chronicity of the ulcer was a major factor in prognosis. Palmer (2) has been a strong advocate of early and aggressive use of endoscopy in all patients with upper gastrointestinal bleeding. He reported that a precise diagnosis of the site of bleeding was possible in 93% of 1400 patients by combined use of early endoscopy and barium contrast studies. Similar results have also been reported by Kalm and Smith (17). No dispute exists as to the accuracy of endoscopic diagnosis, but some have questioned whether this precision in diagnosis improves the outcome for a group of patients. Sandlow et al (18) and Morris et al (19), in two randomized prospective studies, have compared outcome in terms of survival and length of hospital stay between patients in whom an aggressive diagnostic approach was used and those in whom a more conventional program was employed. They were unable to demonstrate any differences. Palmer (2), who used endoscopy routinely, reported overall mortality of 7.9%. Schiller at al (3) reported a mortality rate of 8.9% without the regular use of endoscopy. It must be noted that Palmer's series included 18.7% of patients with esophageal varices (2) whereas Schiller had only 2.4% of such patients. Since this group has a worse prognosis, the comparison between the two series is not easy. The data at present do not clearly indicate that a precise diagnosis will improve treatment and, thus, the prognosis of patients with upper gastrointestinal bleeding.

We must, therefore, make a decision in this matter on belief instead of data. If we could select out the patient who will rebleed and thus become a major management problem, we could evaluate the benefits or otherwise of the aggressive diagnostic approach in this group, where a priori it may be beneficial. We favor early panendoscopy for patients with upper gastrointestinal bleeding. This preference is based on the following considerations:

1. Palmer has shown that 40% of his patients were bleeding from a site other than that suspected on clinical and radiological grounds (2).

2. Knowledge of the precise site of bleeding can save the surgeon precious time in those patients coming to emergency surgery for recurrent or continuing hemorrhage.

3. Knowledge of the precise site of bleeding is helpful in determining optimal therapy in high-risk patients, such as the elderly or those with serious intercurrent illness.

4. Future treatment of the patient with a previous bleeding episode will be predicated on a knowledge of the true origin of the previous bleed and of the present source.

If panendoscopy is performed, a precise diagnosis is possible in 90% of patients (17). Once this is established appropriate therapy can be instituted, as we discuss in Chapter 5. If, however, endoscopy fails to demonstrate the bleeding site, the question of selective angiography will again have to be considered. The decision for or against this procedure will depend on the patient's condition, on whether there is clinical evidence of continuing bleeding, and the suspected diagnosis (see Chapter 3).

In those patients where circulatory status is unstable (Chapter 4), resuscitative measures will be instituted as indicated. If these measures prove successful and the patient's condition is stabilized, investigations may proceed as discussed above. If gastric lavage has proved effective, endoscopy may be undertaken. Alternatively, one may proceed with angiography and possibly intraarterial vasopressin infusion (Chapter 3). Endoscopy may then be used later if necessary to further define the nature of the bleeding site.

In patients whose circulatory state remains unstable, an immediate decision must be made whether emergency surgery should be undertaken or whether selective mesenteric arteriography should first be attempted. This decision is based on several considerations. First will be the urgency of the situation. If, in the physician's judgment, the patient's condition is so precarious that the time involved in obtaining the arteriograms is too great, immediate surgical intervention is appropriate. This will be particularly true if the clinical data give the provisional diagnosis a high degree of probability and thus indicate the likelihood of successful surgical control of the bleeding site. Clearly, if the diagnosis is of a surgically not correctable lesion (e.g., Osler-Weber-Rendu syndrome), continued conservative measures are indicated. If the clinical data do not allow one to make a reasonably secure diagnosis, and an angiography facility is available, arteriography offers not only the opportunity of identifying the site of bleeding, but also of controlling it, at least temporarily, and thus allowing for more effective restoration of the patient's circulatory status. These decisions involve considerations of many facets of the patient's condition. Thus the patient's age, cardiovascular status in regard to presence or absence of vascular disease in the extremities, and pulmonary status will enter into the decision. The decision should be made in concert by the entire team responsible for the patient's case.

In all patients with gastrointestinal hemorrhage an evaluation of clotting function should be obtained as soon as possible. As shown in Table 2-2, disorders of hemostasis may lead to massive or lesser degrees of bleeding from the digestive tract. Correction of these disorders is often possible by intravenous, or intramuscular, administration of clotting factors or vitamin K, and this can prevent major intraoperative problems. The diagnosis of disorders of clotting function is discussed further in the third section of this chapter (Occult Gastrointestinal Bleeding).

Melena

Upper gastrointestinal bleeding, as indicated, may present without hematemesis, but with passage of black, tarry, loose stools or melena. As illustrated in Scheme 2-2, the process of evaluation of the patient with this presentation will proceed along lines very similar to that discussed in relation to hematemesis. There are, however, some special considerations in these patients.

As in the case of patients presenting with hematemesis, the first step is the evaluation of the circulatory status of the patient. If this is unstable, attention must be paid to restoration of circulatory volume before further investigative steps are undertaken (see Chapter 4). Massive intestinal hemorrhage, however, does not often present with melena alone. Schiff, Stevens, Shapiro, and Goodman (20) showed that when more than 1000 ml of blood was infused over 30 to 60 minutes into the stomach of volunteers, red blood was passed per rectum 4 to 17 hours later. Melena was seen when 100 to 200 ml of blood was infused. Blood is generally considered to be a potent stimulant of intestinal motility. Thus, when large amounts of blood are present in the gastrointestinal tract, passage is rapid and the blood is passed in an unaltered state. However, since a relatively small hemorrhage, with melena only, may be the first sign of a major bleeding episode, intravenous fluids should be started and the necessary blood studies should be obtained as in the patient with hematemesis. Surgical and other appropriate consultation should be obtained.

Confirmation of upper gastrointestinal bleeding

The next consideration must be to prove that bleeding is indeed coming from the upper gastrointestinal tract. As a general rule, true melena is most likely to come from a lesion in this area. However, it has been demonstrated that melena may occur when the bleeding site is in the lower ileum or the cecum. Thus Luke, Lees,

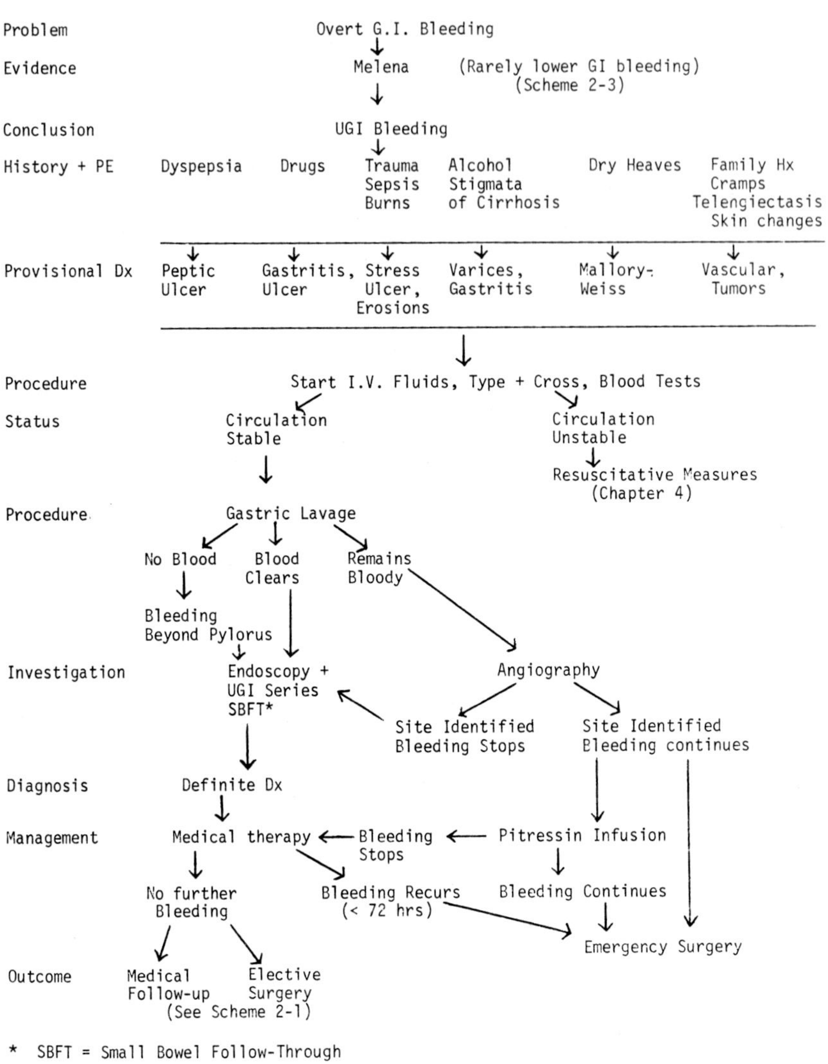

SCHEME 2-2

and Rudick (21) showed that when 25 to 400 ml of outdated bank blood is introduced into the cecum at the time of laparotomy, melena may occur depending on the time taken for the blood to appear in the stool. This observation was confirmed in unoperated subjects by Hilsman (22), who showed, however, that melena was unusual when blood was introduced into the cecum in normal volunteers. Therefore, whether this would occur in normal clinical practice is uncertain. Indeed, Luke et al (21) indicate that melena is rare in colonic bleeding. In patients with hemorrhage from a Meckel's diverticulum (23) the stool is usually red or dark red. On the other hand, lesions in the upper small bowel may well present with melena. Schiff and colleagues (20) observed melena after introduction of 100 to 200 ml of blood into the stomach. With volumes of 1000 ml or more, red blood was seen in the stool after 4 hours, followed by melena some 20 hours later (20). It is noteworthy that stools remained positive for occult blood for 5 to 12 days in some patients (20). This aspect is discussed further in Chapter 5. We may, therefore, conclude from these studies that melena most likely is a feature of upper gastrointestinal bleeding, but it may occur with bleeding lower down if passage of the stool is much delayed. By contrast, rapid passage of blood from upper digestive tract hemorrhage may yield red blood in the stool.

Therefore, further steps must be undertaken to demonstrate the upper gastrointestinal tract origin of the hemorrhage in patients presenting with melena. The first simple, and quick, method is the insertion of a nasogastric tube for aspiration of gastric content. The presence of blood in the aspirate clearly confirms the impression of upper gastrointestinal hemorrhage. This blood may be red or altered (coffee ground) in appearance. The presence of occult blood in the gastric aspirate, in the absence of frank blood, is suggestive, but not conclusive, evidence for an upper digestive tract origin of bleeding, since the trauma of suction and passage of the tube may produce mild bleeding. Another useful indicator of the source of bleeding is the blood urea nitrogen. Schiff and Stevens (24) demonstrated in 1939 that an elevation of BUN over 40 mg per 100 ml in the face of a serum creatinine of less than 1.5 mg per 100 ml, suggested an upper gastrointestinal hemorrhage of more than 1000 ml. With blood loss of similar magnitude from the distal small bowel or cecum, elevation of BUN does not occur. Melena, in the absence of hematemesis, especially when recurrent, suggests bleeding from the distal duodenum or small intestine (25,26). Thus McHardy et al (26) reported that 21 of 46 patients with small-bowel lesions causing overt hemorrhage had melena, and that 69% had a history of previous hemorrhage or anemia.

Provisional diagnosis

Once the clinical determination has been made as to the probable site of origin of the hemorrhage, the provisional diagnosis can be established as in the case of patients presenting with hematemesis. Table 2-1 shows the major causes of upper gastrointestinal hemorrhage, while Table 2-2 lists some of the less frequent etiologies. The clinical means of arriving at a provisional diagnosis have been discussed under the first section of this chapter (Upper Gastrointestinal Bleeding) dealing with hematemesis. The possibility of a bleeding site distal to the proximal duodenum must be borne in mind in these patients. This is especially true in those patients in whom the gastric aspirate is free of blood. Such patients, particularly if there is a past history of melena or anemia, should be evaluated with a high index of suspicion for the rarer causes of bleeding listed in Table 2-2.

A careful clinical search for evidence of vascular and connective tissue disease is mandatory, since these diagnoses depend on the clinical findings (Table 2-2). The mucus membranes should be carefully searched for telengiectasia both at the time of admission, and again after restoration of circulatory volume. These lesions are small arteriovenous fistulae and may close when the patient is hypovolemic. McHardy et al (26) found that small-bowel lesions accounted for about 2% of overt gastrointestinal hemorrhages. These lesions account for a higher proportion of cases of recurrent anemia or melena without hematemesis. McHardy et al (26) reported that 24 of 46 patients with bleeding small-bowel lesions had malignant tumors, while 11 were bleeding from a Meckel's diverticulum and 6 from benign tumors. Identification of these lesions requires very careful clinical evaluation and radiological investigation.

Investigation

The investigation of the patient with melena will proceed as for patients with hematemesis (see preceding section). If the gastric aspirate contains blood, lavage should be performed. If this is successful, and the returns become clear, upper gastrointestinal endoscopy is performed in patients whose condition is stable, and may identify the source of bleeding. If, however, gastric lavage fails to clear the stomach, consideration should be given to undertaking selective mesenteric angiography as a means of identifying the source of hemorrhage (see Chapter 3). In patients in whom the gastric aspirate is free of blood, the bleeding site is presumed to be beyond the pylorus. Panendoscopy may again identify the causative lesion, if it is in the first or second part of the duodenum. If no lesion is seen, the question of angiography must again be considered. Since the localization of a bleeding site by angiography depends on active bleeding at a rate of 0.5 to 2.0 ml per min at the time of study, the chances of identifying the site of bleeding are best during active bleeding. Barium contrast studies may then be performed for further confirmation.

In patients whose condition is unstable when first seen, first priority is given to resuscitative measures (Chapter 4). If these prove successful, investigation may then proceed as described above. If, however, the condition of the patient remains unstable, a decision must be reached, as in the case of patients with hematemesis, whether immediate surgical treatment is indicated, or whether angiography should first be undertaken. These considerations have been discussed in Section 1 above.

LOWER GASTROINTESTINAL BLEEDING

Red Rectal Bleeding (Scheme 2-3)

The patient who presents with passage of bright red or dark red blood per rectum is generally presumed to be bleeding from the distal small bowel or colon. This presumption will prove to be justified in the great majority of cases. Rarely a patient with massive bleeding from a lesion in the stomach or proximal bowel will present with red blood per rectum (20,22). In this case, however, there is usually clinical evidence of massive blood loss, as well as elevation of the BUN. By contrast, massive hemorrhage from the lower intestine is relatively rare. Thus Noer and colleagues (27), in a review of 245 patients with rectal bleeding seen over a 5-year period, found that only 10% were classified as severe, that is requiring transfusion. Only a few of these were massive. Seventeen of the 24 patients in the severe category were found to be bleeding from diverticular disease. Welch and Hedberg (28) stated that only 5% of patients with bleeding from diverticular disease seen at the Massachusetts General Hospital required surgical treatment.

Provisional Diagnosis (Table 2-3)

Major causes of rectal bleeding (red blood) are shown in Table 2-3, together with an indication of their major features and relative frequency. In the majority of these patients (27,28) bleeding will be mild to moderate and, therefore, clinical evaluation and investigation may proceed as indicated in Scheme 2-3.

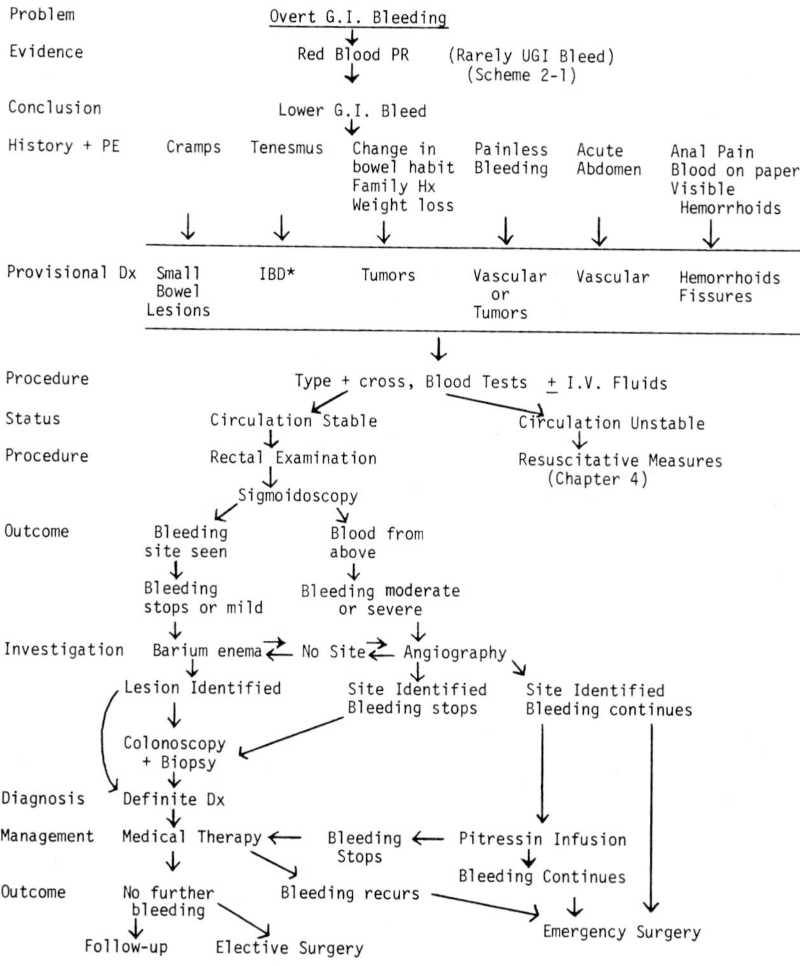

SCHEME 2-3

Carcinoma of the colon. This condition is most commonly seen in patients over the age of 40. Bleeding from malignant tumors of the colon and rectum is usually mild or occult. In one series, only 3 of 89 patients required transfusion (27). If the lesion is in the left colon the major symptoms are of change in bowel habit, with alternating diarrhea and constipation and sometimes tenesmus. The majority of these lesions are within reach of the sigmoidoscope (29). When the tumor is in the right colon, presentation is often asymptomatic, or with weight loss and tiredness related to anemia. Physical findings may include an abdominal mass often due to retained fecal material proximal to the tumor. The liver may be enlarged suggesting possible metastatic involvement. Rectal examination is an essential part of the evaluation, and may reveal the diagnosis if the lesion is in the rectum.

Table 2-3
Major Causes of Lower Intestinal Bleeding

Disease	*Cardinal Features*	*Age*	*Frequency**
Carcinoma of left colon	Change in bowel habit Diarrhea and constipation Cramps	>40	75/245 (27)†
Diverticular Disease			
Right-sided	Commonly asymptomatic	>50	78/245 (27)†
Left-sided	Diarrhea or constipation Cramping pain		70% right sided (31)
Inflammatory bowel disease			
Ulcerative colitis	Bloody diarrhea Tenesmus, weight loss	10-70	39/245 (27)†
Crohn's disease	Diarrhea, weight loss Perianal disease	10-70	Rarely severe
Polyps	Diarrhea, occasional cramps	Any	25/245 (27)†
Carcinoma of right colon	Painless bleeding, anemia, diarrhea	>40	14/245 (27)†
Other causes			

Small bowel tumors	Abdominal cramps	Any	Rare, but about 50%
			  of small bowel
			  bleeds (26)

Meckel's diverticulum	Usually painless	<25	Rare (23)
Vascular malformations	Usually asymptomatic Small bowel or right colon	Any	Rare (34,35)
Bowel infarction	Acute surgical abdomen— small bowel or colon	>50	Rare
{Hemorrhoids	Anal pain, red	Any}	Rare cause of
{Anal fissures	blood in small amounts	Any}	major bleeding

*Numbers in parentheses refer to references.
† Reference 27—A study of 245 patients with bleeding from the colon.

Diverticular disease. Diverticular disease of the colon is an extremely common condition that affects up to 30% of people over 60 years of age (30). Therefore, it is a lesion that is very likely to be found in patients evaluated for intestinal bleeding. Major bleeding as a complication of diverticular disease has been reported to occur in less than 5% of such patients in a number of large series (31,32,33). Proof that it is the cause of bleeding must be, therefore, sought on the basis of positive findings rather than on the basis of exclusion. Recently, by use of selective arteriography, it has been claimed that in more than 70% of patients with diverticular disease and major hemorrhage, the bleeding site is in the right colon (34,35). Further studies in larger groups of patients are necessary to confirm this observation. Nevertheless, angiography should be considered prior to surgery in these patients. Major hemorrhage is more likely to occur in patients with so-called diverticulosis than in those with diverticulitis (26). Therefore, most patients presenting with significant rectal bleeding due to diverticular disease will have few symptoms of bowel disease. Lesser degrees of hemorrhage may well occur with diverticulitis, however. Patients with diverticulitis commonly complain of left lower quadrant pain, cramping, and either constipation or diarrhea. Physical examination will often show tenderness over the inflamed bowel, and a palpable mass may be present. Rectal examination may reveal blood on the examining glove and tenderness.

Inflammatory bowel disease. Ulcerative colitis and Crohn's disease may present with rectal bleeding. These two conditions may affect people at any age, but most commonly start in the second or third decade of life. *Ulcerative colitis* usually presents with bloody diarrhea, tenesmus, often accompanied by fever and weight loss. The bleeding is rarely massive, but because of chronic blood loss anemia is common. There may be extracolonic manifestations of the disease with arthritis, clubbing, uveitis, or erythema nodosum. Perianal lesions, such as fissures or fistulae, occur in about 20% of patients (36). Physical examination is often limited to evidence of weight loss, extracolonic manifestations, and bloody stool or mucous on rectal examination. *Ulcerative proctitis* may be clinically indistinguishable from colitis, but patients with proctitis usually show fewer systemic signs of their disease. *Crohn's disease* rarely presents with major rectal bleeding. Indeed, only about 16% of patients with granulomatous bowel disease show overt bleeding (37). Diarrhea is generally less severe than with ulcerative colitis. However, perianal lesions are very common, being found in about 80% of patients with colonic involvement. Physical examination, therefore, may show perianal abscesses or fistulae, as well as other extraintestinal findings, as in colitis. Rectal examination will often reveal blood, and may show evidence of a perirectal abscess.

Colonic polyps. Polyps in the colon may be single or several *adenomatous lesions, villous adenomata,* or be multiple as in *familial polyposis* or *Gardener's syndrome.* Bleeding from these lesions is rarely massive. However, diarrhea and anemia, due to chronic blood loss, are common. Physical findings are usually limited to finding polyps on rectal examination, except in Gardener's syndrome where soft tissue and bony tumors especially of the head are classically present. Since familial polyposis and Gardener's syndrome are potentially malignant processes, a careful search for evidence for metastatic spread, such as hepato-megaly, is mandatory.

Other causes. *Small bowel tumors* and *Meckel's diverticulum* account for about 2% of cases of intestinal hemorrhage (25,26). The bleeding is often recurrent and over half the patients have a history of previous bleeding episodes or anemia. They may complain of midabdominal cramping pain. Physical examination is generally unrevealing. Patients with *vascular malformation* also commonly present with a history of previous bleeding episodes with no definitive diagnosis as to source. Physical examination may show vascular lesions in the buccal or nasal mucosa or in the rectum. *Angiodysplasia* of cecum and right colon has recently been well documented by Baum (34,35). This lesion occurs primarily in older patients (over 50), often with hypertensive heart disease or aortic valve disease (38). Thus this lesion should be considered in patients with hypertension or aortic stenosis, and angiography should be undertaken if no other cause of bleeding is discovered. *Bowel infarction* may cause severe rectal bleeding. Infarction may be due to occlusion of the *superior mesenteric artery* or *vein.* In this case, the patient presents with severe abdominal pain, and evidence of an acute surgical abdomen. The cardinal finding is bleeding in the face of a silent abdomen. Most commonly this catastrophe complicates advanced atherosclerosis or polycythemia rubra vera, but it may also be *embolic* in origin. This latter possibility should be borne in mind in patients with valvular heart disease or atrial fibrillation or both, since embolectomy may be possible with salvage of the bowel if carried out promptly. Occlusion of the *inferior mesenteric artery* often occurs gradually and silently because of good collateral circulation from the middle colic and hemorrhoidal vessels. However, if it occurs acutely, the presentation is with rectal bleeding, and severe lower abdominal pain, suggesting an acute abdominal catastrophe. This usually happens in elderly patients with arteriosclerotic heart disease. It is important to remember that the rectum is usually spared because of arterial blood supply via the hemorrhoidal vessels. *Hemorrhoids* and *anal fissures* rarely cause massive bleeding. On the rare occasions that they do so the diagnosis is readily made on direct inspection of the perineum.

Procedure

As indicated in the preceding discussion, massive bleeding from the lower bowel causing shock is rare. Therefore, in most patients further evaluation can proceed as is outlined in Scheme 2-3. In the rare instances where circulatory embarrassment is present, resuscitation will be necessary (see Chapter 4). The usual blood studies (Hgb, Hct, serum electrolytes, BUN, typing and crossmatching, prothrombin time, and platelet count) should be obtained and, if clinically indicated, intravenous fluids, including blood replacement, should be started. Vital signs and urine output should be monitored. Once these steps have been initiated, a rectal examination should be performed. In a few instances this will reveal the likely causative lesion, such as a rectal carcinoma. If the rectal examination shows the rectum to contain blood, but no fecal material, and the patient's status permits, we believe sigmoidoscopy should be undertaken forthwith. If the rectum is full of stool, sigmoidoscopy will have to await appropriate cleansing of the bowel. The type of cleansing procedure to be undertaken will have to be determined in the light of the provisional clinical diagnosis. Thus, for example, in patients believed to have acute ulcerative colitis or diverticulitis, enemas and strong laxatives must be used with great caution.

If, however, the rectum is sufficiently clear for sigmoidoscopy, this procedure will yield very valuable information. In patients with recent hemorrhage we prefer to perform this examination in the left lateral decubitus position, since this imposes less stress on the patient. The first question to be answered by the examiner is whether bleeding is occurring from the rectum, or whether blood is coming from above. Local lesions such as fissures and hemorrhoids will have been identified by inspection of the perineum. The lesions that may be seen in the rectum include carcinoma, polyps, or proctitis. In ulcerative colitis or proctitis, the rectal mucosa is uniformly edematous, velvety red, friable and may show ulcerations or pseudopolyposis. In Crohn's disease, the rectal mucosa may resemble that seen in colitis, or may be normal, or show patchy proctitis. If the patient's condition permits and the examiner is experienced, a biopsy of any lesion seen should be obtained for confirmation of the diagnosis.

If the rectal mucosa is normal, but blood is seen coming from above the instrument further studies will need to be undertaken to identify the site of bleeding. The choice will then have to be made as to whether barium contrast studies, such as barium enema, or arteriography should next be undertaken. This decision should be made in the light of the presumptive clinical diagnosis, and in consultation with the surgical consultant. Colonoscopy is another useful diagnostic modality in such patients, but it cannot be performed until the bowel has been fully cleansed, which takes 2 to 3 days. Thus this procedure is usually reserved for later evaluation of lesions suspected following radiologic studies.

OCCULT GASTROINTESTINAL BLEEDING (SCHEME 2-4)

Evidence

Occult bleeding as defined in Chapter 1 is evidenced by the presence of blood in the stool on chemical tests, when it is not evident on gross inspection of the feces. The first necessity, therefore, is to establish the criteria for determining the presence of blood in the stool. Second, it must be established that this blood, if present, is of endogenous origin. These two requirements are, however, not easily met. There is still a good deal of uncertainty as to the best test for establishing the presence of blood in feces. The benzidene test has been shown to be very sensitive, indeed, so much so as to be of questionable value clinically. Three other tests are presently in general use: namely, the guaiac test, hematest tablets©, and hemoccult© slides. Ostrow and colleagues (39) have attempted to evaluate these tests in volunteers given Cr^{51} labeled red cells intragastrically. By using the fecal loss of Cr^{51} as a reference, they found that with the guaiac and hematest procedures, 49% and 27% respectively of stool samples yielded false positive reactions. The hemoccult test gave no false positive reactions, but with this test there was a 50% incidence of false negative reactions. Furthermore, there was significant observer variation in reading the results with all three tests. At the present time, therefore, it is clear that no test is really satisfactory. It is most important that the clinician be familiar with the limitations of the procedures he or she chooses to use. Thus the clinician should know to what extent ingestion of red meat might affect the test being used. Benzidene and guaiac are sensitive enough to detect 1 to 2 ml of blood taken this way, but the others are unlikely to give positive reactions under these conditions. There are conflicting data in the literature on the effect of oral iron and of vitamin C on these various tests. The former may result in false positive tests, while the latter may produce false negative results. In view of these considerations, it is essential that a positive test be confirmed by repeated testing, or by other clinical data, before it is accepted as an indication for an extensive gastrointestinal evaluation.

Presentation

The patient with occult bleeding from the digestive tract will usually present with symptoms of:

1. The underlying disease, for example, heartburn in esophagitis or cramping lower abdominal pain in diverticular disease.

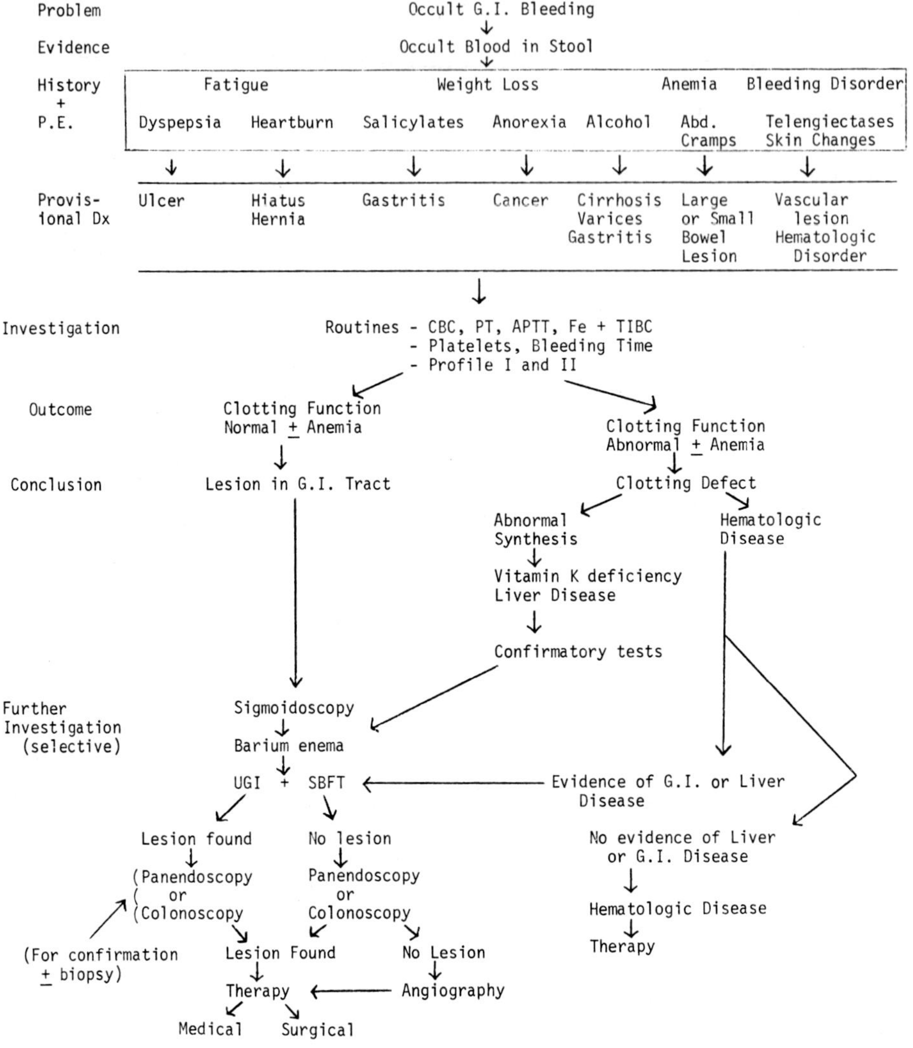

SCHEME 2-4

2. Fatigue and malaise due to the anemia resulting from blood loss.

3. Weight loss, anorexia, or other nonspecific symptoms due, perhaps, to a carcinoma.

Thus, in contrast to patients with overt hemorrhage, the presenting symptoms do not necessarily point to the digestive tract as the source of the problem in patients with occult bleeding. It may be only the finding of a positive test for occult blood in the stool which directs the physician's attention to the digestive tract.

Provisional Diagnosis

All the conditions discussed previously under hematemesis, melena, and rectal bleeding may cause occult bleeding (Tables 2-1, 2-2, and 2-3). The patient may give a history suggestive of one of these lesions. For example, complaints of epigastric pain in bouts and relieved by food or antacids, would suggest peptic ulcer. Heartburn with or without dysphagia indicates esophagitis usually due to a hiatal hernia. A history of prior gastric surgery should raise the possibility of marginal ulcer or gastritis. Gastric carcinoma often presents with anorexia and weight loss, while carcinoma of the colon often leads to altered bowel habit. Particular attention should be paid to a careful inquiry as to ingestion of medications that contain salicylates (12,13). Croft and Wood (40) showed that 70% of 226 subjects taking aspirin had positive tests for occult blood, sometimes with measured losses of as little as 2 ml daily. Therefore, in patients who take even a few salicylate tablets daily, whether it be for minor symptoms or by prescription, for example, for rheumatoid arthritis, stool tests should be repeated after discontinuation of salicylates for 2 to 3 days. If under these conditions the stools become negative for occult blood, it is likely that the bleeding is drug induced. For confirmation, the cycle should be repeated. This simple maneuver may save the patient many time-consuming and expensive investigations.

Investigation

The first step in evaluating a patient with occult bleeding as shown in Scheme 2-4 should be a hematologic screen including a complete blood count, red cell morphology, platelet count, bleeding time, pro-thrombin time, and activated partial thromboplastin time. The purpose of these studies is to determine whether the blood loss has been sufficient to result in anemia, or whether there is an underlying hematologic disorder. If anemia is present and red cell morphology suggests hypochromia, a determination of serum iron and iron-binding capacity may be obtained for confirmation of iron deficiency. Moreover, the combination of bleeding time, platelet count, prothrombin time, and partial thromboplastin time will detect the clinically significant clotting defects of more than 90% of patients (41). As a further part of the routine screening procedure, it is useful to obtain blood for serum electrolytes, blood sugar, BUN, serum proteins, albumin, cholesterol, calcium, creatinine, alkaline phosphatase, bilirubin, and transaminase. These studies are used to screen the patient for major metabolic disorders, such as uremia, for evidence of liver disease, or protein losing enteropathy (e.g., inflammatory bowel disease), which may be the cause of gastrointestinal bleeding. Abnormalities in any of these screening tests may dictate special tests for their further elucidation.

Defects in clotting function are often suggested by the clinical history. For example, patients with hemophilia or Christmas disease are usually males with a typical family history and episodes of recurring massive bleeding. Idiopathic thrombocytopenia purpura is usually first manifested under the age of 40 years, and is evidenced by the characteristic purpuric lesions in most cases. Von Willebrand's disease is suggested by finding of a prolonged bleeding time in a patient with a normal platelet count. Defects in clotting function should also be considered in all patients thought to have liver disease. However, clotting defects require confirmation by means of laboratory investigation, as is indicated at the beginning of this section. Table 2-4 summarizes these screening tests and the significance of the abnormalities noted. The bleeding time is prolonged in patients with platelet deficiency, or impaired platelet aggregation or adhesion. Therefore, abnormality in this test will direct attention to platelet disorders. Heavy salicylate ingestion can produce such effects, as can other anti-inflammatory drugs, such as Indomethacin or Phenylbutazone, and should be considered. This is unusual, however, in therapeutic dosage. A prolonged prothrombin time is frequently seen in patients with liver disease, or patients with malabsorption of vitamin K due to either small-bowel disease, or biliary obstruction. In the latter two instances, parenteral administration of vitamin K results in rapid correction of the abnormality. Of particular significance, for diagnosis, is the finding of a normal prothrombin time in the face of a prolonged activated partial thromboplastin time. This finding indicates a deficiency of factor VIII, IX, or XI and thus suggests hemophilia, or Christmas disease if the clinical setting is appropriate.

When evidence of clotting disorder has been obtained, a determination must be made whether this is due to a defect in synthesis of clotting factors as seen in liver disease, or vitamin K deficiency, or whether the problem results from a hematologic disorder. In the presence of clinical evidence of liver disease, the hepatic origin of the clotting problem is strongly supported by finding a low level of factor V. Vitamin K deficiency is suggested by a history of diarrhea or steatorrhea, or obstructive jaundice. In such patients there is deficiency of factors II, VII, IX, and X, which together with the prothrombin time promptly respond to vitamin K therapy.

Many hematologic disorders can result in bleeding disorders due to platelet abnormalities, or deficiencies of clotting factors. Such disorders will be suggested by the clinical history and findings, as indicated, in many instances. The screening tests will often provide additional diagnostic information. Full elucidation will require complete hematologic evaluation. In this group of patients further evaluation of the gastrointestinal tract may be postponed unless clinical or

Table 2-4
Tests of Clotting Function*

Test	*Significance of Abnormality*
Bleeding time	Prolongation indicates platelet disorder
Prothrombin time (PT)	Prolongation indicates decrease in Factors I, II, V, VII, and X
Activated partial thromboplastin time (APTT)	Prolongation indicates abnormalities of factors I, II, V, VIII, IX, X, XI, XII
PT normal APTT prolonged	Deficiency of factors VIII, IX and XI

*(See Reference 41)

laboratory data indicate the presence of significant disease in the digestive tract, which requires attention in its own right. The proper sequence of studies then should be worked out in consultation with the hematologist.

If the clinical history and physical findings suggest a primary disease of the gastrointestinal tract, and clotting function has been shown to be normal, it is likely that the source of blood loss is in the digestive tract. Further examination will then be directed to the identification of the likely source of hemorrhage. The precise sequence of investigations will be dictated by the clinical data, and the provisional diagnosis based on them. Some general guidelines are, however, useful. In older patients, in particular, it is best to evaluate the entire digestive tract since more than one lesion may be present, and if so, it will be necessary to determine which is the one responsible for the problem at hand. Saint's triad of diverticular disease, hiatus hernia, and gallstones is a well-known illustration of this axiom. We, therefore, recommend that investigation start with a sigmoidoscopy, and be followed by a barium enema and an upper gastrointestinal series with small-bowel follow-through examination. Upper and lower intestinal fiberoptic endoscopy has two major roles in this group of patients. First, it can provide confirmation visually, or by biopsy, of any lesion shown by radiologic studies. Second, it may reveal lesions not demonstrable by barium contrast examination. We discuss these aspects in more detail in Chapter 3.

One of the more troublesome problems in the management of a patient with occult gastrointestinal bleeding is the definitive identification of the bleeding site. All the lesions listed in Tables 2-1, 2-2, and 2-3 may cause occult bleeding. Since many of them are common disorders, which are often incidental findings, the physician must seek clear evidence that the bleeding is indeed coming from that lesion. *Hiatus hernia* is a good example of a very common disorder. Inglefinger (42) has estimated that it occurs in up to 50% of elderly individuals. Others have suggested that hiatal hernia is found in 30% of patients over the age of 55. However, it has been the experience of many that this lesion is often an incidental finding (15). To establish that a hiatal hernia found during radiologic evaluation is the cause of hemorrhage, there should be clinical evidence of gastroesophageal reflux and esophagitis, that is, regurgitation and heartburn. The clinical impression must be supported by either a positive Bernstein test (acid perfusion) (43) or the finding of esophagitis, with a friable esophageal mucosa, at endoscopy, or both.

Diverticular Disease is another common finding in older patients. It is very difficult to prove that this lesion is the source of bleeding. Even when the patient has symptoms suggesting that the diverticular disease is clinically significant, it may not be the source of blood loss. Thus Rigg and Ewing)31), in reviewing this problem, found that mild bleeding was reported in 5% to 40% of cases, while Bolt and Hughes (32) in a series of 100 patients found minor bleeding to be very common. On the other hand, Birke and Engstedt (44) reported no bleeding in a series of 163 cases of diverticulosis of the colon. We believe that if the patient has lower abdominal pain, a mass with definite tenderness over the bowel, and no other lesion demonstrated, it is reasonable to assume that the diverticular disease is the source of bleeding. However, such patients should be followed closely, and if bleeding persists, colonoscopy should be undertaken to be sure that an underlying carcinoma is not missed.

Peptic ulcer and *esophageal varices* are generally considered as causes of overt gastrointestinal bleeding. No data exist to our knowledge as to how often these lesions are responsible for significant occult bleeding. When either of these lesions is the only abnormality detected in this clinical setting after full evaluation, including panendoscopy, it may be presumed to be the source of bleeding. Careful follow-up is mandatory. In the case of peptic ulcer, bleeding should stop with medical therapy. Persistent bleeding should raise suspicion of malignancy, especially in patients with gastric ulcer, or of another lesion, and such bleeding should be fully reinvestigated with endoscopy, biopsy, and cytology. In patients with esophageal varices, persistent occult bleeding presents a particularly difficult problem. If bleeding is of sufficient magnitude (0.5-2 ml/min), angiography should be undertaken. However, in this case endoscopy will usually have made the diagnosis. Clotting function must be fully evaluated, and if necessary, the gastrointestinal tract must be examined endoscopically and radiologically. If

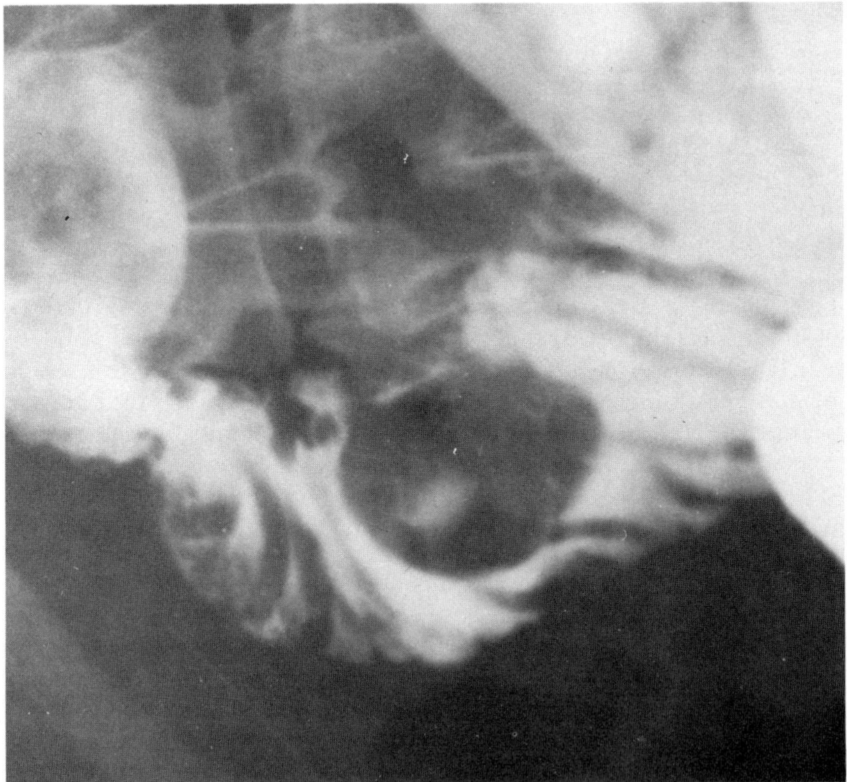

FIGURE 2-1   LEIOMYOMA OF DUODENUM
Radiograph of descending portion of duodenum shows large circular
filling defect due to the tumor, with a collection of barium slightly above
the center. This latter represents the ulceration commonly seen in this type
of tumor. The patient, a 16-year-old girl presented with recurrent
episodes of painless melena.

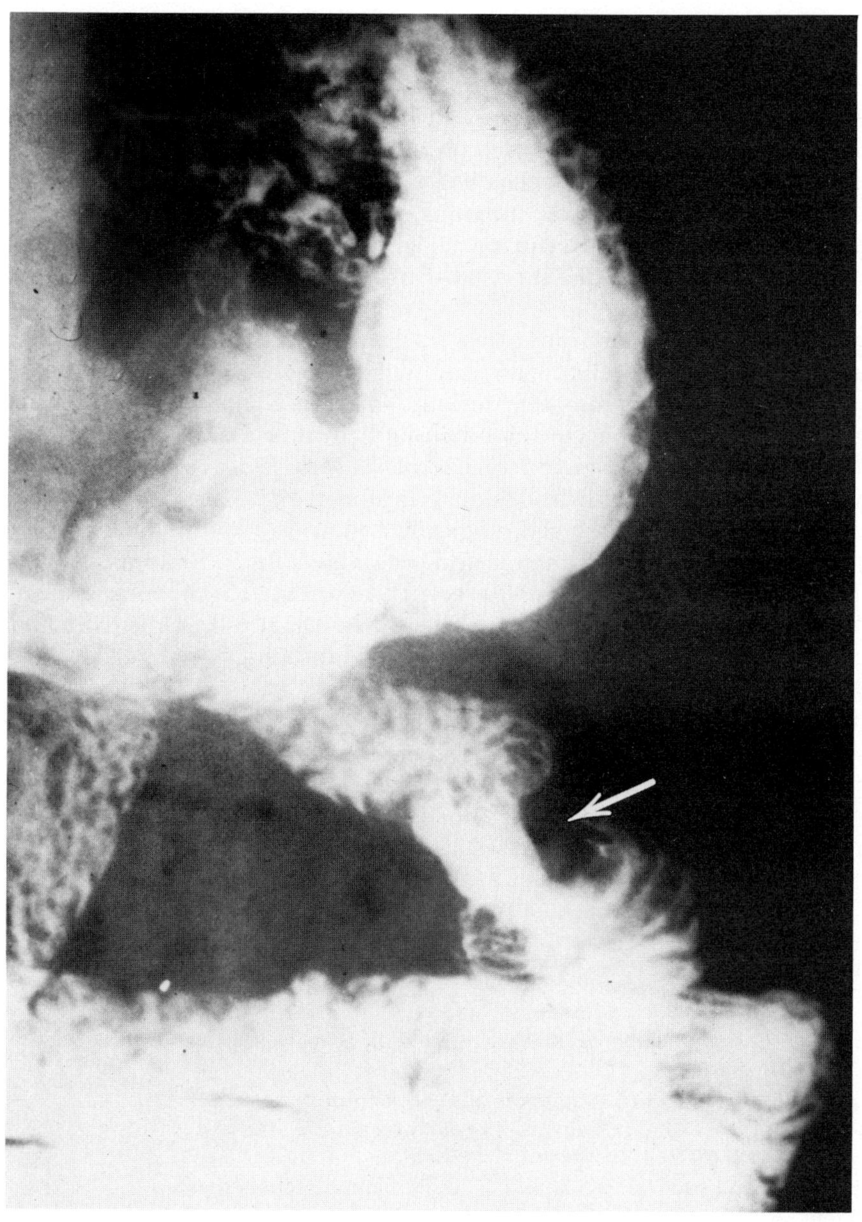

FIGURE 2-2   ADENOCARCINOMA OF JEJUNUM
In the jejunum just beyond the ligament of Treitz there is a narrowed
area (arrow) where the mucosal pattern is effaced at site of the carcinoma.
This study is from a 56-year-old lady with repeated episodes of severe iron
deficiency anemia.

again, no other lesion is detected, and the blood loss is clinically significant, the question of surgical therapy may need to be considered (Chapter 5).

The approach to patients with a history of *salicylate ingestion* has already been discussed. It is a very common cause of occult bleeding. Proof that salicylates are the cause of the problem is based on retesting the feces after withdrawal of the medication, and subsequent rechallenge if indicated. Upper gastrointestinal endoscopy can help further to confirm the diagnosis. This procedure may also reveal *gastritis* due to other causes. In general, gastritis should only be accepted as a cause of hemorrhage if friability or mucosal hemorrhages are seen at endoscopy.

Malignant tumors of the gastrointestinal tract commonly present with anemia secondary to occult bleeding. Characteristically, bleeding once started is persistent unlike the case with inflammatory lesions, where it is intermittent. Hence, persistently positive tests for occult blood should prompt a careful search for tumors of the digestive tract (Figure 2-1). *Carcinoma of the fundus of the stomach* or *cecum* may present this way with few other symptoms, and must, therefore, be looked for with special care both radiologically and endoscopically. *Small-bowel tumors* (26) may also present with anemia and occult bleeding. This lesion should be suspected particularly in patients with recurrent anemia. Sometimes cramping midabdominal pain will suggest the diagnosis. Diagnosis is difficult and requires careful, and perhaps repeated, small-bowel radiology (Figure 2-2). Angiography may show a tumor blush (Chapter 3).

Detailed family history and careful physical examination will usually help establish a diagnosis in patients with *hereditary telengiectasia, pseudoxanthoma elasticum,* and *Ehlers-Danlos syndrome* (Table 2-2). Indeed, these diagnoses will rarely be missed, despite their rarity, if they are borne in mind during examination of a patient, since the physical findings are so striking.

REFERENCES

1. Major, R. H.: *Classic Descriptions of Disease.* 3rd Ed., Blackwell, pp. 628–632, Oxford, 1955.
2. Palmer, E. D.: The vigorous diagnostic approach to upper gastro-intestinal tract hemorrhage. A 23-year prospective study of 1400 cases. *JAMA,* **207:**1477, 1969.
3. Schiller, K. F. R., Truelove, S. C., and G. D. Williams: Hematemesis and melena, with special reference to factors influencing outcome. *Brit. Med. J.* **2:**7, 1970.
4. Mallory, G. K., and Weiss, S.: Hemorrhage from lacerations of the cardiac orifice of the stomach due to vomiting. *Amer. J. Med. Sci.* **178:**506, 1929.
5. Saylor, J. L., and Tedesco, F. J.: Mallory-Weiss syndrome in perspective. *Amer. J. Digest. Dis.* In press.
6. Harkins, H. N.: Acute ulcer of the duodenum (Curling's ulcer) as a complication of burns, relation to sepsis. *Surgery,* 1939.
7. Mears, F. B.: Autopsy survey of peptic ulcer associated with other disease. *Surgery,* **34:**640, 1953.
8. Beil, A. B., Mannix, H., and Beal, J. M.: Massive upper

gastro-intestinal hemorrhage after operation. *Amer. J. Surg.* **108:**324, 1964.

9. Breckenridge, I. M., Walton, E. W., and Walker, W. F.: Stress ulcers in the stomach. *Brit. Med. J.* **2:**1362, 1959.

10. Finer, D. I., and Fry, J.: Peptic ulcer in general practice. *Brit. Med. J.* **2:**169, 1955.

11. Hanscom, D. H., and Buchanan, E.: The Veterans Administration Cooperative Study of G.U.—Chapter 4, The Follow-up Period. *Gastroenterology,* **61:**585, 1971.

12. Alvarez, A. S. and Summerskill, W. H. J.: Gastrointestinal hemorrhage and salicylates. *Lancet,* **1:**920, 1958.

13. Winkelman, E. I.: Salicylates and the G.I. Tract—A review. *Univ. Mich. Med. Bull.* **26:**182, 1960.

14. Jones, F. A.: *Modern Trends in Gastroenterology.* Butterworth and Co., Ltd., London, 1952.

15. Jones, F. A. and Gummer, J. W. P.: *Clinical Gastroenterology.* Blackwell, Oxford, 1960.

16. Lewin, D. C. and Truelove, S.: Hematemesis with special reference to chronic peptic ulcer. *Brit. Med. J.* **1:**383, 1949.

17. Kalm, R. M., and Smith, F. W.: Panendoscopy in the early diagnosis of upper gastrointestinal bleeding. *Gastroenterology,* **65:**728, 1973.

18. Sandlow, L. J., Beeker, G. H., Spellberg, M. A., Allen, H. A., Berg, M., Berry, L. H. and Newman, E. A.: A prospective randomized study of the management of UGI hemorrhage. *Amer. J. Gastro.* **61:**282, 1974.

19. Morris, D. W., Levine, G. M., Soloway, R. D., Miller, W. T., and Marin, G. A.: Prospective randomized study of diagnosis and outcome in acute upper gastro-intestinal bleeding: Endoscopy versus conventional radiography. *Amer. J. Digest. Dis.* **20:**1103, 1975.

20. Schiff, L., Stevens, R. J., Shapiro, N., and S. Goodman: Observations on oral administration of citrated blood in man—Effect on stools. *Amer. J. Med. Sci.* **203:**409, 1942.

21. Luke, R. G., Lees, W., and Rudick, J.: Appearance of the stools after the introduction of blood into the cecum. *Gut,* **5:**77, 1964.

22. Hilsman, J. H.: The color of blood containing feces following instillation of citrated whole blood at various levels of the small intestine. *Gastroenterology,* **15:**131, 1950.

23. Rutherford, R. B., and Akers, D. R.: Meckel's diverticulum—A review of 148 patients with special reference to the pattern of bleeding and to mesodiverticular vascular bands. *Surgery,* **59:**618, 1966.

24 Schiff, L., and Stevens, R. J.: Elevation of urea nitrogen content of the blood following hematemesis and melena. *Arch. Intern. Med.* **64:**1239, 1939.

25. Segal N. L., Scott, W. J. M., and Watson, J. S.: Lesions of the small intestine producing massive hemorrhage. *J. Amer. Med. Assoc.* **129:**116, 1945.

26. McHardy, G., Bechtold, J. E., and McHardy, R. J.: Hemorrhage from primary disease of the mesenteric small intestine—Review of the literature and analysis of 216 cases. *Gastroenterology,* **28:**17, 1955.

27. Noer, R. J., Hamilton, J. E., Williams, D. J., and Broughton, D. S.: Rectal hemorrhage: Moderate and severe. *Ann. Surg.* **155:**794, 1962.

28. Welch, C. W., and Hedberg, S.: Gastrointestinal hemorrhage, I. General considerations of diagnosis and therapy. *Adv. Surg.* **7:**95, 1973.

29. Copeland, E. M., Miller, L. D., and Jones, R. S.: Prognostic factors in carcinoma of the colon and rectum. *Amer. J. Surg.* **116:**875, 1968.

30. Manousos, O. N., Truelove, S. C., and Lumsden, K.: Prevalence of colonic diverticulosis in general population of Oxford area. *Brit. Med. J.* **2:**762, 1967.

31. Rigg, B. M., and Ewing, M. R.: Current attitudes to diverticulitis with particular reference to colonic bleeding. *Arch. Surg.* **92:**321, 1961.

32. Bolt, D. E., and Hughes, L. E.: Diverticulitis: A follow-up of 100 cases. *Brit. Med. J.* **1:**1205, 1966.

33. Broders, C. N.: Bleeding from diverticula of the colon. *Surg. Clin. North America,* **52:**315, 1972.

34. Baum, S., Alhanasoulis, C. A., and Waltman, A. C.: Angiographic diagnosis and control of large bowel bleeding. *Dis. Colon and Rectum,* **17:**447, 1974.

35. Baum, S., Athanasoulis, C. A., Waltman, A. C., and Rug, E. J.: Gastrointestinal hemorrhage, II. Angiographic diagnosis and control. *Adv. Surgery,* **7:**149, 1973.

36. Edwards, F. C., and Truelove, S. C.: The course and prognosis of ulcerative colitis. *Gut,* **4:**299, 1973; **5:**1, 1974.

37. *Crohn's Disease,* Brooke, B. W. (ed.), W. B. Saunders Co., London, Philadelphia, 1972.

38. Cody, M. C., O'Donovan, T. P. B., and Hughes, R. W.: Idiopathic gastrointestinal bleeding and aortic stenosis. *Amer. J. Digest. Dis.* **19:**393, 1974.

39. Ostrow, J. D., Mulvaney, C. A., Hansel, J. R. and Rhodes, R. S.: Sensitivity and reproducibility of chemical tests for fecal occult blood with an emphasis on false positive reactions. *Amer. J. Digest. Dis.* **18:**930, 1973.

40. Croft, D. N. and Wood, P. H. N.: Gastric mucosa and susceptibility to occult gastro-intestinal bleeding caused by aspirin. *Brit. Med. J.* **1:**137, 1967.

41. Roberts, H. R. and Cederbaum, A. I.: The liver and blood coagulation: Physiology and pathology. *Gastroenterology.* **63:**297, 1972.

42. Ingelfinger, F. J.: *In Principles of Internal Medicine.* Harrison, T. R., Adams, R. D., Bennett, I. L., Resnick, W. H., Thoru, G. W., and M. M. Wintrobe (eds.), 4th Edition, McGraw-Hill Book Co., New York, 1962.

43. Bernstein, L. M., and Baker, L. A.: A clinical test for esophagitis. *Gastroenterology,* **34:**760, 1958.

44. Birke, G., and Engstedt, L.: Melena and hematemesis—A follow-up investigation with special reference to bleeding of unknown origin. *Gastroenterologia,* **35:**97, 1956

3
DIAGNOSTIC METHODS: ENDOSCOPY AND ANGIOGRAPHY

In the preceding chapters the definitions of the types of gastrointestinal bleeding are discussed together with the modes of presentations of various causative disease states. Here we consider the various diagnostic modalities available to the physician for the full evaluation of the patient with gastrointestinal bleeding.

As we stress in the preceding chapters, the initial cardiovascular resuscitation must precede any prolonged diagnostic procedures. Of equal importance is the need for the combined efforts of the appropriate specialists. The initial evaluation may be made by a primary care physician, internist, or surgeon but, if they are available, the team should include an endoscopist and an angiographer as well. The resources of each of these specialists should be committed to the patient's care, when and if the physician primarily responsible for the patient's care deems appropriate. Although current data do not seem to indicate any decrease in mortality with the vigorous diagnostic approach, at our institution we prefer to approach the problem of gastrointestinal bleeding in the manner we have described. The reasons for this preference have already been stated in Chapter 2. Specifically, the future treatment of a patient with gastrointestinal bleeding will be determined by an absolute anatomical diagnosis, for example, a bleeding duodenal ulcer, as may be the case in patients with cirrhosis with varices who present with hematemesis. It has been well shown that as many as 30% to 60% of cirrhotics with known varices and upper gastrointestinal bleeding, have lesions other than the varices as the source of their blood loss (1,2,3). Thus in a patient who presents with hemorrhage, early use of endoscopy or angiography may show the bleeding to be due to gastritis, whereas later investigation may show only esophageal varices which, however, were not the cause of bleeding. Therefore, although the mortality may not have changed since the advent of the vigorous diagnostic approach, it is our feeling that appropriate, specific management of most patients will depend on an absolute anatomic diagnosis. Not only will the decision for or against surgery often be made on the basis of specific investigations such as endoscopy or angiography, but the timing of that intervention, and the time it takes, may be altered by previous diagnostic maneuvers. In retrospect, Cruveilhier's patient would have benefited from angiography to document the anatomic site of bleeding, perhaps pitressin infusion to diminsh or stop blood loss and permit cardiovascular resuscitation, and finally definitive surgical therapy.

The value of gastric aspiration has already been mentioned. By this technique, one wishes only to document the presence, or absence, of fresh, or partially digested blood. Mention should be made of the possibility of inducing artefactual lesions in the gastric mucosa, which may confuse later endoscopy. The longer the tube is left in place, the more artefacts will be created; furthermore, the tube may produce irritation of a lesion already present, for example, a Mallory-Weiss tear. Therefore, once the presence, or absence of blood has been verified, and if necessary, and possible, the stomach lavaged, the tube should be removed. The other two universally available diagnostic tests, the rectal examination with testing of the stool for blood, and the sigmoidoscopic examination have also been discussed in the preceding chapters.

Radiological examinations of stomach, duodenum, small bowel, and colon are well-established methods for defining potential sources of bleeding in the gastrointestinal tract. This approach to diagnosis in the patient with acute hemorrhage has some major limitations. First, as will be shown later, barium x-ray examination cannot be relied on to demonstrate some common sources of upper gastrointestinal bleeding such as hemorrhagic gastritis or Mallory-Weiss tears (Table 3-1), since these lesions are too superficial for radiologic detection. Second, even when a lesion, such as a peptic ulcer, is documented by radiography, this does not prove that that lesion is the source of bleeding. Yet a decision for or against surgical treatment of a patient with a radiologically demonstrated lesion and bleeding cannot be made with confidence without knowing whether that lesion is responsible for the hemorrhage. Finally, the presence of barium in the intestinal tract can prove a serious hazard to a patient who requires an emergency operation. The barium may become inspissated in the bowel leading to intestinal obstruction, stercoral ulceration, and even bowel perforation.

The revolution in the diagnostic approach to bleeding from the gastrointestinal tract has come with the availability of panendoscopy and angiography. These procedures supplement, but do not necessarily replace the usual barium examinations. The first two procedures have been used enthusiastically to define the exact source(s) of bleeding in most cases. Recent reports have indicated that precise diagnosis was possible in as many as 97% of patients with upper gastrointestinal bleeding (4,5), using the modern flexible endoscopes capable of panendoscopy, that

Table 3-1*

Lesions Seen	*On Endoscopy*	*By X-ray*	*Percent of Dxs Made by X-ray*
Esophagitis	31	1	3
Gastritis	85	3	3.5
Mallory-Weiss	28	1	3.5
Duodenal ulcer	287	126	44
Gastric ulcer	96	36	37.5
Esophageal varices	23	13	56.5
Gastric carcinoma	12	8	67
Totals	562	188	33.5%

*(Data summated from studies by Cotton, Sugawa, Classen, and Katon) (4,5,10,11).

is, esophago-gastroduodenoscopy, including retroflexion for careful inspection of the cardia and the gastroesophageal junction from below.

PERORAL PANENDOSCOPY

In our institution we prefer to evaluate the patient as early as possible, even in the emergency room. As noted in the decision trees, the unstable patient not responding to volume and red cell replacement must be taken to the operating room or the angiography suite, and is not a candidate for endoscopy. The patient who continues to bleed profusely as shown by the stomach tube drainage cannot be examined unless the blood is removed. An efficient way of accomplishing this is to pass an Ewald tube into the stomach and lavage assiduously with saline, except in the patient with cirrhosis where caution should prevail because of the danger of sodium overload. If the return from the stomach can be cleared, immediate endoscopy can be performed. If the drainage remains grossly bloody, we forego endoscopy in favor of angiography. In Palmer's study (6) of some 1400 patients, he used similar techniques and reported only 87 examination failures secondary to inadequate visualization; and it must be remembered he used a nonmalleable endoscope. The endoscope used today is usually an end-viewing instrument, as opposed to the oblique or side-viewing endoscope. However, the oblique viewing instrument can be utilized, and may in some instances give a better view of the channel and parts of the duodenal bulb. The earlier that the procedure is done following the acute bleeding episode the better are the chances of positive identification of the bleeding site. Endoscopy is most particularly useful in the recognition of inflammatory lesions such as gastritis or esophagitis. Other lesions, such as the Mallory-Weiss tear or an ulcer in a hiatal hernia, are also notoriously hard to define by barium studies.

Another indication for endoscopy may, in the near future, be for therapeutic intervention. Endoscopic hemostasis has either been accomplished or is being contemplated by methods such as laser photocoagulation, cryocoagulation, suture clip placement, and tissue "glues." These methods are, however, still in the experimental stage and are awaiting full evaluation for efficacy and safety.

The contraindications for panendoscopy are relatively few. The most important factors, of course, are the clinical state of the patient, and the experience and expertise of the endoscopist. Assuming that both are acceptable to the physician responsible for the patient, the following relative contraindications should be kept in mind.

1. Acute myocardial infarction. Endoscopy may precipitate arrhythmias. Serious arrhythmias (e.g., trigeminy, frequent multifocal PVC's, etc.), themselves may constitute a contraindication.

2. Acute respiratory distress. Even patients without pulmonary disease sometimes find it hard to "breathe around the tube" and, in addition, intravenous diazepam may act as an acute respiratory depressant. This last effect may be seen especially in older patients.

3. A combative, uncooperative patient, or one in delerium tremens. Under these circumstances, endoscopy is unlikely to be rewarding, and may be more

hazardous with a higher likelihood of adverse effects from the procedure (see below).

4. Tracheal intubation. This may present difficulty in passage of the endoscope, and may be a factor in esophageal perforation. Some proceed with endoscopy without change in technique despite the endotracheal tube, although Sugawa et al deflated the cuff until the endoscope was passed and then reinflated it (5).

5. Suspected or proven perforation of a peptic ulcer or bowel infarction.

6. Other conditions that may predispose to complications, such as esophageal perforation, include severe cervical spine arthritis or esophageal diverticula, especially a Zenker's diverticulum.

The preparation of the patient is relatively simple. After the initial cardiovascular resuscitation has been achieved, the pharynx is anesthetized with a spray or gargle of topical anesthetic. Intravenous diazepam is used to achieve a suitable state of sedation and amnesia, bearing in mind the profound vascular effects that this drug may have, especially in this setting. It is helpful to pass an Ewald tube before the endoscope for several reasons: (1) it allows the endoscopist to feel his way about the posterior pharynx with a very soft tube before inserting the more rigid, albeit malleable endoscope; (2) it gives the endoscopist a "dry run" in which he can assess the patient's reaction to a large-bore tube being passed through the mouth and upper esophageal sphincter; (3) it allows for emptying of the stomach and evaluation of its contents, as well as lavage of the stomach as mentioned above.

An experienced endoscopist who performs the procedure at an appropriate time in the patient's course can do so with a very low morbidity rate. In a recent report (7) on endoscopy, using data collected in a retrospective study, the mortality of esophagoscopy alone varied from 0.06% to 0.003%, while perforation and bleeding occurred in 1/1000 and 1/1500 patients, respectively. In gastroscopic examina-

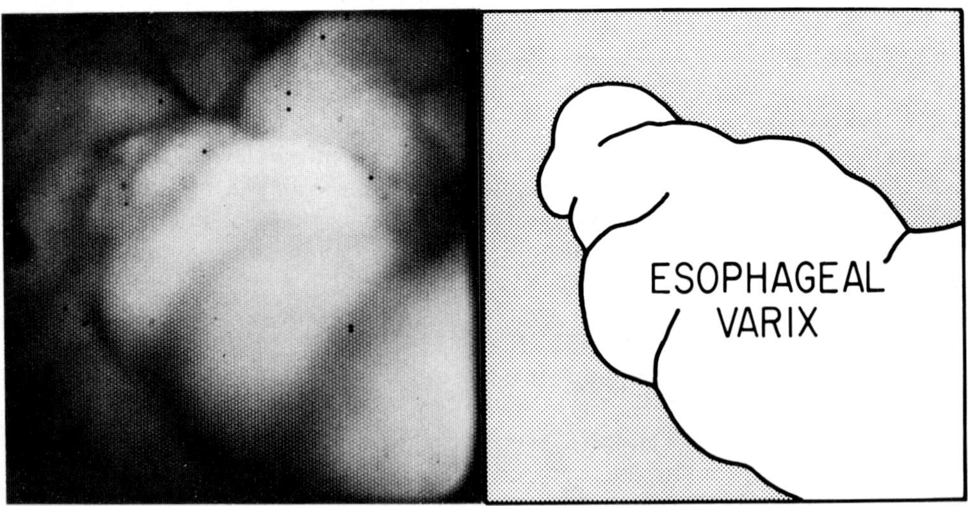

FIGURE 3-1
Endoscopic photograph of large esophageal varices in a patient presenting
with history of excess alcohol ingestion and melena. No other lesion was found
at the time of examination, at which time bleeding had stopped.

tions the rate of perforation was 1.2/1000. Duodenoscopy, of course, included the above procedures and the morbidity rate was 1.4/1000. In the more than 211,000 upper gastrointestinal endoscopies reviewed over a period of time spanning several generations of instruments, there were 70 perforations, 36 bleeding episodes after biopsy, 129 cardiopulmonary problems, 17 infections, and 128 miscellaneous adverse reactions, for a total complication rate of 1.32/1000. Adverse reactions from sedatives, mainly cardiovascular changes, respiratory depression, and occasionally paradoxical agitation may occur, especially in the elderly. Occasionally an experienced endoscopist may wish to "talk the scope down," but we believe it is advisable to produce short-term amnesia with intravenous diazepam so as to make the procedure more comfortable and acceptable to the patient. This is particularly important in those patients whose lesion may require follow-up evaluation by repeated endoscopy.

It has been clearly shown that the diagnostic yield of endoscopy decreases with increasing time between the bleeding episode and the examination. Forrest (8) successfully identified the bleeding site in 78% of his patients when they were examined within the first 24 hours. Positive diagnosis of the bleeding lesion was achieved in only 60% of cases examined 48 hours after the bleed and in only 32% of those examined more than 48 hours later. More recent studies (5) have reported success rates as high as 97% when the examinations were done early, and with modern instruments. In Palmer's classic study (6), 33.4% of diagnoses were first made by the upper gastrointestinal radiography that immediately followed esophagogastroscopy. However, one should remember that Palmer used the older rigid instruments, which did not permit visualization of the gastric fundus or the duodenum. Finding multiple lesions at the time of endoscopy is a common experience. In Sugawa's (5) study, 43% of patients had a second bleeding site. Knauer (9) showed that 83% of patients with a Mallory-Weiss lesion had a second mucosal abnormality, most commonly in the stomach. Comparisons of the diagnostic accuracy of endoscopy as against radiological examination would be easier to evaluate if endoscopists routinely obtained photographic documentation of their findings. Endoscopic photography is readily accomplished with modern instruments and is valuable in providing documentation of the lesions seen. Four recent studies comparing the two modalities are summarized in Table 3-1. It is evident that modern endoscopy is more consistently fruitful than a barium study, especially in the first three categories, namely esophagitis, gastritis, and the Mallory-Weiss tear.

COLONOSCOPY

Colonoscopy permits full examination of the lower bowel, but to be successful it requires vigorous preparation. Generally, patients are given a liquid diet for 24 to 48 hours before the procedure, and they need extensive cleansing enemas to assure unimpeded visualization of the colonic mucosa. Colonoscopy has, therefore, a limited role in the diagnostic evaluation of the acute lower gastrointestinal bleeder, the most valuable tool here being angiography. There are, however, some reports of attempts at colonoscopy in this setting. Schmitt et al (12) studied 9 such cases and succeeded in visualizing a source of bleeding in 2 of them (splenic flexure ulcer and vascular ischemia); but none of the 9 were bleeding massively at the time. Deyhle et al (13) examined 18 patients with acute hemorrhage from the colon. They localized a bleeding site within the colon in 15, and excluded a colonic site in 2. Despite enemas immediately before colonoscopy, they found the mucosa still obscured in places by feces and clotted blood, but were able to wash this away during the examination. In fact, 6 cases were treated via the colonoscope, 3 were treated with diathermy snare of bleeding polyps, 2 other post-polypectomy bleeding sites were treated with diathermy coagulation, and 1 hemangioma, also with a diathermy snare. None of these patients required angiography or surgery. This report is encouraging, but the findings need confirmation, before this approach can be generally recommended.

The greatest role for colonoscopy is in the patient with chronic lower intestinal bleeding, especially when the barium enema is negative or nondiagnostic.

Relative contraindications to colonoscopy are acute colonic inflammatory bowel disease, large aortic or iliac aneurysm, recent pelvic or colonic surgery, pelvic adhesions, pregnancy, severe ischemic bowel disease, acute irradiation colitis, peritonitis, or an uncooperative patient. It should be emphasized that these contraindications are relative, not absolute. The risks involved are directly related to the experience of the colonoscopist, and they consist basically of perforation and/or bleeding. Smith and Nivatvongs (14) sent questionnaires to 32 physicians in the United States, Japan, and England, who were known to do large numbers of colonoscopies. The 22 who responded reported a total of 7959 procedures. Of those, 6290 were done for diagnositc purposes with 7 complications for a rate of 0.1%. In the 1669 polypectomies, there were 48 complications, for a rate of 2.9%. Somewhat higher figures come from a recent review under the auspices of the National Institute of Arthritis, Metabolism and Digestive Disease (15). In 25,298 examinations there were 50 perforations, 23 bleeding episodes, 10 cardiopulmonary complications, 3 infections, and 15 miscellaneous adverse reactions. The overall morbidity was 3.46/1000.

Sedation of the patient, as with upper gastrointestinal endoscopy, is achieved with intravenous diazepam with or without meperidine. Although some colonoscopists utilize fluoroscopy during the procedure, many do not. Here the experience and preference of the endoscopist is paramount. The decision whether to use colonoscopy in the evaluation of the patient with lower intestinal bleeding must be based on a knowledge of the risks of the procedure and its potential for providing a precise diagnosis, and thus a basis for definitive therapy.

A study of Shinya and Wolff (16) is of particular interest in this regard. In this study they reported 125 cases with both barium enema and colonoscopic examinations. There were 31 cases with a negative or questionable barium enema, with a positive colonoscopic examination. The most frequently found lesion was a polyp, 17 of them being 0.5 to 2.0 cm in diameter. The recent literature (17,18) favors colonoscopy as the diagnostic tool of choice for the patient with chronic rectal bleeding. The air contrast technique for examination of the colon might provide a better diagnostic yield than the routine barium enema, but it is not used routinely, because it is considered potentially dangerous by some radiologists. Colonoscopy is still a relatively new procedure, and a final decision on its role in the evaluation of patients with presumed colonic bleeding must await future studies. At present, we do not advocate colonoscopy in the acute bleeder, preferring angiography. In the patient with a past history of lower intestinal bleeding, we do a barium enema first, and then follow at a later date with colonoscopy if there is doubt as to the diagnosis.

ANGIOGRAPHY

With the advent of the Seldinger femoral catheterization technique, which replaced the translumbar approach, abdominal angiography has become a much more useful, and more frequently used, technique for evaluation of the gastrointestinal bleeder. As we mentioned previously, accurate and specific diagnosis requires knowledge of the precise site of bleeding, and angiography is well suited to this goal. In addition to precise localization, angiography offers the prospect of an increasingly wide range of therapeutic interventions (see Chapter 5).

Angiography is indicated for patients with upper gastrointestinal bleeding in whom endoscopy is not possible for any one of the reasons discussed earlier, or in whom intraarterial infusion therapy (see Chapter 5) is being considered. In the patient with lower intestinal bleeding one may wish to proceed immediately with angiography. However, since many episodes of hematochezia cease spontaneously, and the patient never deteriorates clinically, some physicians may choose to support the patient and wait. If bleeding stops, angiography need not be done. If it persists, angiography should be made available.

If the bleeding is defined as coming from the upper gastrointestinal tract, the angiographer will first inject the celiac artery. Although selective catheterizations of this type are frequently unrewarding because they do not permit visualization of the bleeding site, they do allow the angiographer to define the specific vascular anatomy in that particular patient. When this has been done, the catheterization can then be made superselective, that is, by cannulation of the left gastric artery for the majority of the stomach, of the right gastric artery for the antrum, and of the gastroduodenal artery for the duodenum. If the bleeding site is still not identified, the superior mesenteric artery (SMA) should be catheterized and injected. If a bleeding site exists distal to the proximal duodenum (e.g., a tumor of the jejunum), this study may allow a diagnosis to be made. In the patient with esophageal variceal bleeding an injection of dye into the SMA will document angiographically the presence of varices. The dye injected into the SMA traverses the splanchnic bed, and is returned via the splenic and mesenteric veins, and thence into esophageal varices, should portal hypertension be present. The dilution of dye that occurs during this transit does not prevent visualization of the varices, but does make it very unusual to see extravasation of dye, that is, a "bleeding" varix. Therefore, the angiographic diagnosis of bleeding esophageal varices is established by the lack of demonstration of an arterial or capillary bleeding site, and the presence of varices (see Figure 3-1). Endoscopy should be attempted if possible, to confirm that the esophageal varices are the source of bleeding, before one makes the definitive diagnosis with all its implications. For lower intestinal bleeding, both the superior mesenteric artery (SMA) and the inferior mesenteric artery (IMA) should be catheterized and injected. The former supplies the bowel from the ligament of Treitz to the splenic flexure, and the latter supplies the bowel from the splenic flexure to the rectum.

The contraindications to angiography are relative. The patient with an unstable cardiovascular system may be unsuitable for angiographic investigation. However, since angiography may be therapeutic in a dramatic manner (see Chapter 5), some patients who are in the midst of volume resuscitation can be taken to the angiography suite, as long as appropriate arrangements are made for careful patient monitoring while the angiography is under way. A clotting disorder is a second relative contraindication. It must be defined and corrected as rapidly as possible if that is feasible. Such intervention itself may slow bleeding, and it will also decrease the risk of femoral artery puncture and catheterization. However, if the coagulation defect is not correctable, angiography should not be undertaken. The third most important contraindication to this procedure is advanced atherosclerosis, which is present in many of the older patients. As will be discussed, the incidence of complications rises with the presence of severe atherosclerosis, but this lesion itself is not an absolute contraindication. The patient with low output cardiac failure, or previous arterial thrombosis is also at special risk. Lang canvassed 300 physicians about their complication rate, and in 11,402 examinations analyzed, he found 7 fatalities and 81 serious complications for rates of 0.06% and 0.7%, respectively (19). He further reported 3% minor adverse reactions, which included temporary arterial spasm, asymptomatic local hematomas, asymptomatic intramural or subintimal injections, and perforation of a major vessel without sequelae. The serious complications included arterial thrombosis, usually at the site of needle puncture, but occasionally at a distant point probed during catheterization. Forty-seven patients lost a limb as a result of this complication. Other serious effects were arterial emboli, hematomas, pseudoaneurysms, and small-bowel ileus. Manipulation of the catheter, especially in the patient with advanced atherosclerosis, may produce small atheromatous emboli, which may lodge anywhere, but are especially dangerous to the kidneys. The dye itself seems to be relatively well tolerated.

The major advantages of angiography are that patient preparation does not require gastric lavage or cleansing enemas, and the procedure itself, coupled with intraarterial infusion therapy, may help in the resuscitation of the patient. Furthermore, the procedure is done with only local anesthesia at the site of artery puncture.

In the patient with upper gastrointestinal hemorrhage, the procedure has been shown convincingly to be of value in localization of the bleeding site (3,20,21,22,23). The failures usually result from inability to do superselective catheterizations, or the cessation of bleeding prior to the examination. Bleeding must be proceeding at a rate of 0.5 to 2.0 ml per min for visualization to be accomplished. Table 2-1, Chapter 2, lists the major sources of upper gastrointestinal bleeding, that is, peptic ulcer, gastritis, esophageal varices, and Mallory-Weiss tears. All of them may be visualized by the angiographer (Figure 3-2).

The most common causes of massive lower intestinal bleeding are diverticula and vascular malformations. Less frequently massive bleeding may result from carcinoma, inflammatory bowel disease, and polyps. Depending on the clinical impression as to the most likely diagnosis as outlined in Table 2-4 (Chapter 2), either the SMA or IMA may be injected first, although generally the distribution of both are examined. Once again. the bleeding must be active for angiography to be of diagnostic value, except in vascular malformations and some tumors. In an interesting study by Eisenberg et al (24), 7 patients out of 45 had their bleeding site visualized only after repeated injections of contrast material. This may be related to the vasodilating effects of the dye itself. Baum has recently described a disorder he calls angiodysplasia (20,21), which usually presents as painless hematochezia in older patients. The pathologist may have difficulty in demonstrating this lesion in the resected specimen. In fact, these are submucosal vascular lakes which may bleed profusely if the overlying mucosa is disturbed. Of clinical interest is the more frequent localization of these lesions in the colon proximal to the splenic flexure

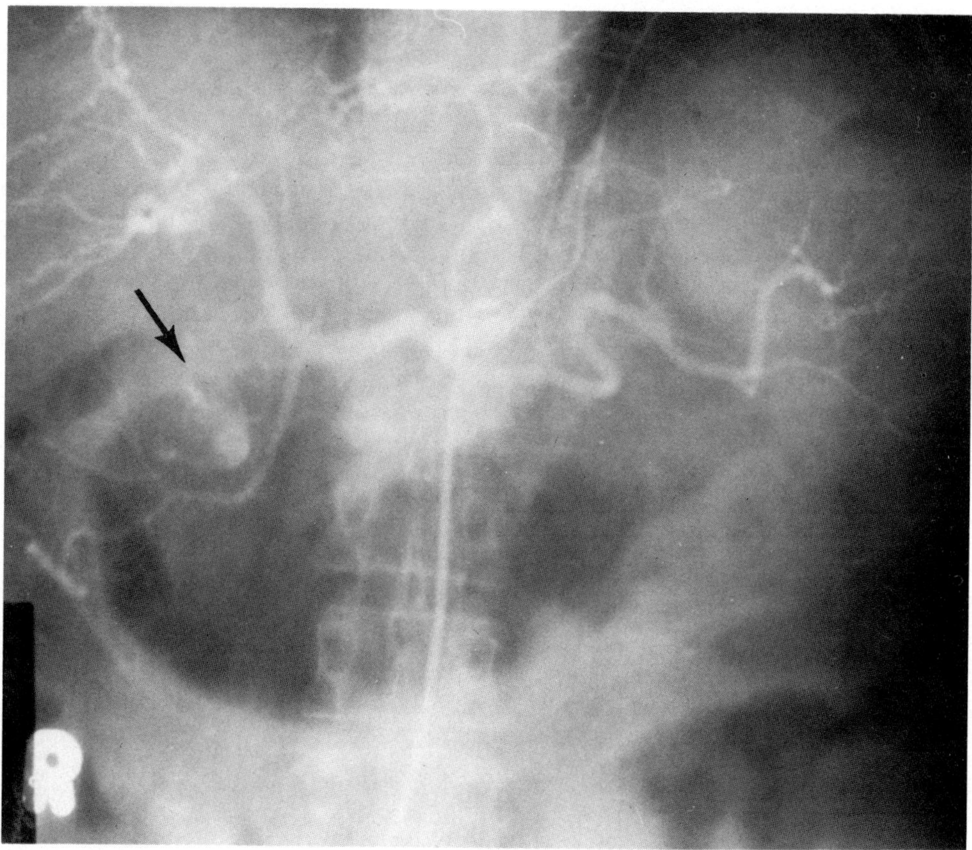

FIGURE 3-2
Celiac artery injection in a patient with documented cirrhosis of the liver and esophageal varices by barium x-ray studies. The patient developed hematemesis in the hospital. Endoscopy could not be done because of continuing bleeding. Angiography demonstrated extravasation of dye into the duodenum (arrow) from a branch of the pancreaticoduodenal artery. Duodenal bleeding was successfully controlled initially by pitressin infusion.

(20,21). This localization has also been demonstrated for bleeding diverticula (24,25,26). However, in the patient who presents with hematochezia and previously documented diverticula, as many as one third may be bleeding from another lesion (26). Any patient who presents with a second bleeding episode from the lower intestinal tract that is separable from the first by a significant time period, for example, several weeks, should undergo repeat angiography. Even if the first episode had a well-documented site of bleeding, one cannot assume a common source.

Direct comparisons of angiography and barium studies are difficult, since the latter examination precludes the use of the first, and many physicians proceed from angiographic diagnosis to arterial infusion therapy and forego barium studies completely. The special and difficult problem of chronic gastrointestinal bleeding will be discussed in Chapter 6, but a study by Sheedy et al (27) is worthy of comment in relation to the value of angiography in this clinical setting. This study embraced 88 patients with chronic bleeding (range 3 months to 22 years). Forty-four had previous surgical procedures, which were neither diagnostic nor curative. Seventy-four of these 88 patients had extensive radiographic and endoscopic evaluations. Despite the absence of active bleeding at the time of angiography, Sheedy et al (27) were able to establish a likely source of bleeding in 45% of these patients. That is, a lesion was identified that was thought to be the previous bleeding site, although it was not actively bleeding at the time. Of the lesions found, one half were arteriovenous malformations, and one half of these were in the cecum or ascending colon. Unfortunately, in the patients with a negative study, two carcinomas (small-bowel and cecum) were later found at surgery.

Angiography has proved its worth in the diagnosis of both upper and lower intestinal bleeding. Once the lesion has been identified, control of bleeding can frequently be accomplished, as we discuss in Chapter 5. At the very least, angiography offers the surgeon the knowledge of the precise site of bleeding and, therefore, allows for more rapid operative management.

REFERENCES

1. McCray, R. S., Martin, F., Amir-Ahmadi, H., Sheahan, D. G., and Zamcheck, N.: Erroneous diagnosis of hemorrhage from esophageal varices. *Amer. J. Digest. Dis.* **14:**755, 1969.
2. Conn, H. O., and Bradoff, M.: Emergency esophagoscopy in the diagnosis of upper GI hemorrhage. *Gastroenterology,* **47:**505, 1964.
3. Ring, E. J., Baum, S., Athanasoulis, C., and Waltman, A. C.: Angiography in the diagnosis and treatment of nonvariceal bleeding in patients with portal hypertension. *Surg. Gyn. Ob.* **139:**205, 1974.
4. Cotton, P. B., Rosenberg, M. T., Waldram, R. P. L., and Axon, A. T. R.: Early endoscopy of esophagus, stomach and duodenal bulb in patients with hematemesis and melena. *Brit. Med. J.* **2:**505, 1973.
5. Sugawa, C., Werner, M. H., Dennis, F. H., Lucas, C. E., and Walt, A. J.: Early endoscopy—a guide to therapy for acute hemorrhage in the upper gastrointestinal tract. *Arch. Surg.* **107:**133, 1973.
6. Palmer, E. D.: The vigorous diagnostic approach to upper gastro-intestinal tract hemorrhage. *J. Amer. Med. Assoc.* **207:**1477, 1969.
7. Work Group X: Instruments for diagnosis, investigation and treatment of digestive diseases. *Gastroenterology,* **69:**1151, 1975.
8. Forrest, J. A. H., Finlayson, N. D. C., and Shearman, D. J. C.: Endoscopy in gastrointestinal bleeding. *Lancet,* **2:**394, 1974.
9. Knauer, C. M.: Characterization of 75 Mallory-Weiss lacerations in 528 patients with upper gastrointestinal hemorrhage. *Gastroenterology,* **71:**3, 1976.
10. Classen, M., Koch, H., and Demling, L.: Duodenoscopy methods and findings. *Gastro. Endoscopy,* **18:**78, 1971.
11. Katon, R. M., and Smith, F. W.: Panendoscopy in the early diagnosis of acute UGI bleeding. *Gastroenterology,* **65:**728, 1973.
12. Schmitt, M. G., Wallace, C. W., Geenen, J. E., and Hogan, W. J.: Diagnostic colonoscopy. *Gastroenterology,* **69:**765, 1975.

13. Deyhle, P., Blum, A. L., Niiesch, H. J., and Jenny, S.: Emergency colonoscopy in the management of the acute peranal hemorrhage. *Endoscopy,* **6:**229, 1974.
14. Smith, L. E., and Nivatvongs, S.: Complications in colonoscopy. *Colon and Rectum,* **18:**214, 1975.
15. Work Group XII: Human experimentation in digestive disease research. *Gastroenterology,* **69:**1165, 1975.
16. Wolff, W., and Shinya, H.: Comparison of colonoscopy and contrast enema in 500 patients with colorectal disease. *Amer. J. Surg.* **129:**181, 1975.
17. Loose, H. W. C., and Williams, C. B.: Barium enema versus colonoscopy. *Proc. Soc. Med.* **67:**1033, 1974.
18. Overholt, B. F.: Colonoscopy, a review. *Gastroenterology,* **68:**1308, 1975.
19. Lang, E. K.: A survey of the complications of percutaneous retrograde arteriography. *Radiology,* **81:**257, 1963.
20. Baum, S., Athanasoulis, C. A., Waltman, A. C., and Ring, E. J.: Gastro-intestinal hemorrhage. Part II. Angiographic diagnosis and control. *Adv. Surgery,* **7:**149, 1973.
21. Novelline, R. A., Waltman, A. C., Athanasoulis, C. A., and Baum, S.: Recent advances in abdominal angiography. *Adv. Int. Med.* **21:**417, 1976.
22. Athanasoulis, C. A., Brown, B., and Shapiro. J. H.: Angiography in the diagnosis and management of bleeding stress ulcers and gastritis. *Amer. J. Surg.* **125:**468, 1973.
23. Reuter, S. R., and Bookstein, J. J.: Angiographic localization of gastrointestinal bleeding. *Gastroenterology,* **54:**876, 1968.
24. Eisenberg, H., Laufer, I., and Skillman, J. J.: Arteriographic diagnosis and management of suspected colonic diverticular hemorrhage. *Gastroenterology,* **64:**1091, 1973.
25. Baum, S., Rosch, J., Dotter, C. T., Ring, E. J., Athanasoulis, C. A., Waltman, A. C., and Courey, W. R.: Selective mesenteric arterial infusions in the management of massive diverticular hemorrhage. *New Engl. J. Med.* **288:**1269, 1973.
26. Casarella, W. J., Kanter I. E., and Seaman, W. B.: Right sided colonic diverticula as a cause of acute rectal hemorrhage. *New Engl. J. Med.* **286:**450, 1972.
27. Sheedy, P. F., Fulton, R. E., and Atwell, P. T.: Angiographic evaluation of patients with chronic gastrointestinal bleeding. *Amer. J. Roent. Rad. Therp. and Nuc. Med.* **123:**338, 1975.

4

HEMORRHAGIC SHOCK

Significant hemorrhage results in widespread systemic adaptations that attempt to restore nutrient supply to immediately vital organs. If, despite these systemic responses, volume depletion is of such magnitude that nutrient flow is unable to support normal cell metabolism, a state of shock supervenes. This state should be suspected when there is tachypnea, tachycardia, hypotension, oliguria, and cutaneous vasoconstriction. (See Scheme 4-1.)

Cardiovascular Responses to Hemorrhage

A sudden reduction in blood volume results in reduced venous return to the heart. The reduced baro-receptor stretch in the carotid sinuses and aortic arch stimulates sympathetic outflow (via the hypothalamus) producing generalized vasoconstriction, sparing the vessels of the heart and brain. Concomitantly heart rate and myocardial contractibility are increased. Clinically, vasoconstriction is most noticeable in the skin, which becomes pale and cool. Hypotension occurs when 30% to 50% of the blood volume has been lost (1).

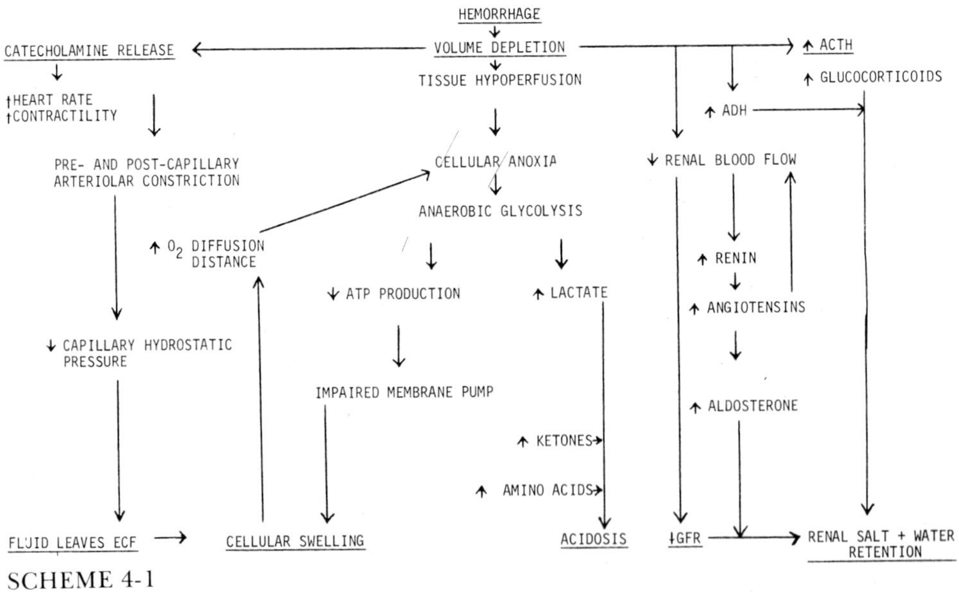

SCHEME 4-1

As a result of adrenergic stimulation, pre- and post-capillary vascular sphincters are constricted in affected areas, and capillary hydrostatic pressure is reduced. Accordingly, based on the Starling hypothesis, fluid moves into the capillaries and tends to restore the intravascular volume (2), at the expense of the extracellular, extravascular fluid space (referred to hereafter as ECF). With more severe hemorrhage, the ECF is further depleted as fluid enters cells that are rendered anoxic by loss of nutrient supply (3). It is thus apparent that in hemorrhagic shock the ECF depletion is greater than would be anticipated from intravascular losses alone (3).

Presumably in response to hemorrhage the ACTH levels are raised, which results in increased output of corticosteroids producing salt and water retention. The major stimulus to salt and water conservation, however, is brought about by renal hypoperfusion and vasoconstriction, causing release of renin. Renin forms angiotensin I and subsequently angiotensin II, which stimulates aldosterone output (4). Finally, in response to ECF reduction, antidiuretic hormone (ADH) is also released, resulting in further water retention by the kidneys.

If hemorrhagic shock continues uncorrected, reduced capillary perfusion results in anoxic tissue metabolism with release of acid metabolites. This produces vasodilatation, with reduction in peripheral resistance. Furthermore, capillary endothelial damage by stagnant anoxia leads to extravasation of intravascular fluid into the tissues. Deterioration of ventricular function occurs in later stages (5) which, coupled with loss of vascular tone, is ultimately the cause of death.

Cellular Metabolic Responses to Hemorrhage

Cellular metabolism is markedly altered by a massive hemorrhage. Reduced tissue perfusion which produces cellular hypoxia favors anaerobic glycolysis. Under these conditions the production of high-energy phosphates such as ATP and creatine phosphate is reduced (6). Schumer has shown interference with conversion of pyruvate to acetyl CoA in primates with hemorrhagic shock (7). The pyruvate formed in anaerobic glycolysis thus accumulates as lactic acid and can be measured in blood as an index of the severity of shock. The lactic acid contributes to the metabolic acidosis of severe hemorrhagic shock. With the loss of energy stores, cellular structural integrity, and hence ionic transport, is compromised. The membrane sodium pump is impaired with entry of water and sodium into the cells and loss of potassium (3). The cells swell (8), and this may cause more intracellular damage because of the increased oxygen diffusion distance from the membrane to inner portions of the cell. Another effect of reduced ATP production may be depletion of intracellular cyclic adenosine monophosphate (cAMP), as demonstrated in experimental hemorrhagic shock (9). It is possible that with progressive depletion of cAMP, response to endogenous catecholamines may be compromised, since these responses are mediated by cAMP.

The adverse role of lysosomal enzyme release in hemorrhagic shock is controversial. It has been postulated that release of acid hydrolases from ruptured lysosomes in anoxic cells may result in shock refractory to treatment (10). These enzymes can hydrolyze microsomal and mitochondrial membranes, reducing oxidative phosphorylation. Thus they lead to further impairment of essential cellular metabolic processes. Further studies are required to demonstrate more directly the damaging effects of lysosomal enzymes in shock. There may well be therapeutic implications in the elucidation of the above hypotheses. Recent experimental studies have suggested some protection from refractory hemorrhagic shock by pretreatment with antiserum to cathepsin D, a potent lysosomal acid protease (11) and with adrenocorticosteroid, which stabilize lysosomal membranes.

Acid-Base Changes in Hemorrhagic Shock

As a result of cellular anoxia in severe hemorrhage, acid-base balance is markedly altered. Most patients with massive hemorrhage develop varying degrees of metabolic acidosis (12). The most obvious explanation is that acidosis is brought about by acid metabolites of anaerobic glycolysis under these conditions. In this regard, it has been shown that lactic acidemia is a sensitive indicator of cellular anoxia (13). Other factors may contribute to the acidosis. Amino acids and nitrogen have been shown to increase in urine following shock (13), indicating a state of catabolism. Increase in the level of circulating amino acids in plasma are presumably secondary to glucocorticoid release. In more severe hemorrhagic shock, the inability of the liver to metabolize the amino acids results in further acidosis. Altered fat metabolism may also contribute to acidosis in hemorrhagic shock. Because of high circulating levels of catecholamines, lipolysis and conversion of triglycerides to free fatty acids in adipose tissue is enhanced. These free fatty acids, when used for ATP production, are metabolized to ketone bodies, which compound the acidosis.

Hyperventilation in milder hemorrhages masks the metabolic acidosis (14). The hyperventilation is presumably mediated through the baro-receptors, or centrally by sympathetic stimulation of the respiratory centers. In severe hemorrhage the increased rate of respiration is not sufficient to compensate, and arterial pH will fall. The severity of acidosis, in fact, may be prognostically significant. Casey et al (15) showed that in a group of patients with hemorrhagic shock mortality was significantly increased in those with arterial pH values less than 7.3.

A moderate degree of metabolic acidosis, however, is not altogether undesirable, since it facilitates release of oxygen and uptake of CO_2 in the tissues. Alkalosis, on the other hand, would tend to have the reverse effect by causing a leftward shift in the oxyhemoglobin dissociation curve (16).

Carbohydrate Metabolism in Hemorrhagic Shock

Hyperglycemia has been observed frequently in shock (17), while insulin levels have been low or normal. Such patients have resistance to the hypoglycemic effects of insulin. It has been postulated that the hyperglycemia and insulin resistance may be related to diminished oxidative phosphorylation in anoxic cells. Catecholamine and glucocorticoid release, however, may also play a role in the production of insulin-resistant hyperglycemia. Despite these obvious reasons, other unknown factors must be involved, since insulin-resistant hyperglycemia persists long after the hormonal changes and tissue anoxia have been reversed (18).

The clinical implications of these observations in the management of patients in shock have not yet been clarified. Theoretically, abnormal glucose utilization by anoxic cells would continue to favor fatty acid and amino acid metabolism to maintain cellular energy stores. These pathways are less efficient than glycolysis in the production of ATP. Attempts to reverse the reduced glucose utilization by administration of hypertonic glucose have resulted in transient improvement in hemodynamic status of patients in severe hypovolemic shock (19). Recent experimental studies have shown also that ATP infusion may reverse insulin resistance in shock (20) by an unknown mechanism. Further studies are needed to determine whether these therapeutic manipulations will improve survival in profound hemorrhagic shock by improving the energy-producing processes in the cells.

Renal Responses to Hemorrhage

Reduction of blood volume results in renal hypoperfusion. Renal blood flow falls in proportion to perfusion pressure and also in response to increased sympathetic activity. Outer cortical blood flow is reduced, with resultant sodium and water conservation secondary to diminished glomerular filtration. The contracted ECF volume further diminishes glomerular filtration. The decreased renal perfusion pressure also enhances output of renin and angiotensin (21), which cause a further fall in cortical flow. With more profound shock the renal medulla is rendered ischemic (22) which, coupled with cortical ischemia, results in tubular cell damage. If volume restoration is delayed, acute renal failure is the outcome; however, this eventuality is rare in situations of pure volume depletion, such as uncomplicated hemorrhage.

Pulmonary Response to Hemorrhage

A syndrome of progressive hypoxia, increasing pulmonary interstitial edema, and lowered pulmonary compliance has been observed frequently in severely injured patients, many of whom died of fulminant respiratory failure (23). Because many such patients were in shock, it was assumed that respiratory failure was secondary to pulmonary ischemia, and the term "shock lung" became popular. It now appears that although hemorrhagic shock alone can produce some pathological abnormalities, such as pulmonary interstitial edema and hemorrhage of varying degrees, progressive hypoxia is not the usual outcome in experimental studies (24). This has been confirmed in clinical studies by Shires (3) where no causal relationship between hemorrhagic shock and pulmonary insufficiency could be established. Nevertheless, increased interstitial pulmonary sodium and water are fairly consistent findings in hemorrhagic shock (17,25), but the significance of this is questionable. The progressive respiratory failure in traumatized patients is probably based on multiple factors, of which shock is only one variable (26).

Treatment *(Scheme 4-2)*

The main objective for treatment of the patient with gastrointestinal hemorrhage is to restore the circulating blood volume as rapidly as possible while instituting measures to control hemorrhage. It is often difficult to estimate the exact volume of blood lost without blood volume determinations, but if a patient manifests the stigmata of shock, it must be assumed that he has lost at least one third of his blood volume rapidly. The end point of therapy is similarly difficult to define, but disappearance of signs of cutaneous vasoconstriction, return of normal pulse and blood pressure, restoration of urine output to over 50 ml per hr, and of hematocrit to

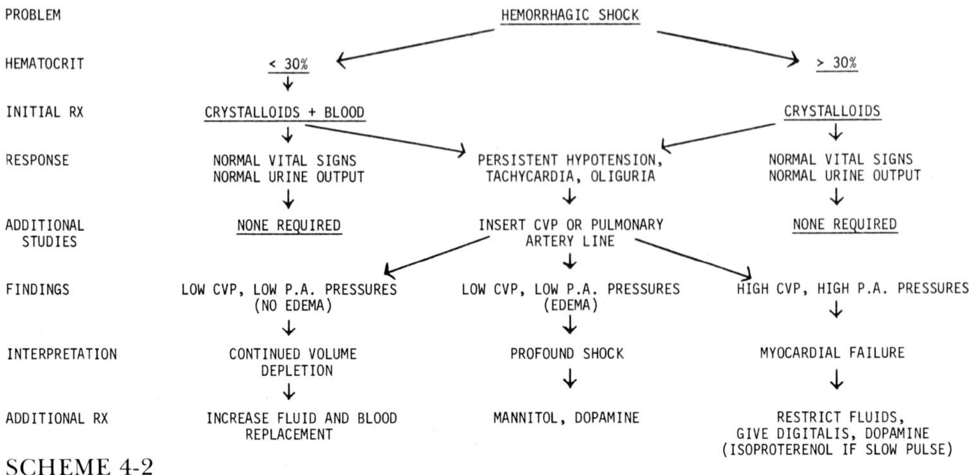

SCHEME 4-2

about 30 volumes% are reasonable guidelines to aim at. Ancillary measurements such as central venous pressure (CVP), cardiac output, blood volume, pulmonary artery, and wedge pressures are extremely useful, if not mandatory, in patients who remain unstable despite seemingly adequate therapy, or who have previous cardiac or renal problems or both. Arterial blood gases and lactate levels are somewhat less invasive studies that can aid in establishing severity of shock and responses to therapy.

EARLY SHOCK

Blood Replacement

The availability of whole blood is becoming increasingly limited because of both practical and therapeutic considerations. Risk of hepatitis can be reduced by administration of packed cells (17). Furthermore, by separating whole blood into respective components of red cells, platelets, and plasma, each can be put into specific use depending on the clinical situation. Despite these considerations, treatment with whole blood is the mainstay for restoration of intravascular volume with continuing hemorrhage.

When blood is being administered in a bleeding patient, several important factors must be taken into account so that its therapeutic benefits are fully realized:

1. Replacement with blood alone is not adequate to restore the disproportionate losses in the extravascular, extracellular fluid space. Experimentally, it has been shown that in dogs, recovery from severe hemorrhagic shock is most rapid when balanced electrolyte solution as well as retransfusion of shed blood is carried out (27). Clinical observations support the contention that replacement of blood alone must be supplemented by electrolyte solutions (28).

2. Massive banked blood transfusions will result in dilution of clotting factors, the more serious being factor V and VII deficiencies. Platelet depletion is not as

frequent a problem, although it has been reported in severe combat casualties (29). The depletion of these factors obviously is dependent on the age and quantity of administered blood. Clotting factor deficits can be treated readily by infusion of fresh frozen plasma and platelets as necessary. Citrate toxicity with massive transfusions is probably rare. Finally, with repeated rapid transfusions, blood should be warmed beforehand because of increased oxygen requirements for maintenance of body temperature if the blood is cold (30).

3. With massive transfusions, microaggregates and cell debris will enter the pulmonary circuit. Older blood has the greatest number of these particles. Although the theoretical harmfulness of these particles on pulmonary function has not been documented fully in clinical situations, the use of micropore filters under these circumstances would seem logical.

4. Stored, aging blood has a progressive increase in hemoglobin-oxygen affinity (31,32), because of a decline in erythrocyte 2,3-diphosphoglycerate. Thus, oxygen delivery to already ischemic areas is further impaired with massive transfusions. This situation can be corrected by use of blood less than three days old when multiple rapid transfusions are anticipated.

Crystalloids and Colloids

In addition to intravascular volume replacement with blood, the extravascular, extracellular volume deficit requires correction. Since balanced salt solutions are readily available, resuscitation can be initiated effectively by their rapid infusion. The crystalloid solutions most frequently used are normal saline or Ringer's Lactate. Hypo-osmolar solutions such as half-normal saline or 5% glucose and water are contraindicated in immediate fluid replacement, since intravascular and ECF fluid losses are isoosmotic. In addition to correction of ECF losses, the administration of crystalloid solutions will reduce the number of transfusions required. It has been estimated that for each volume of whole blood loss, three times as much crystalloid is required for adequate replacement (33). Such a formula, however, does result in some reduction of colloid oncotic pressure, but as long as large enough quantities are used, hydrostatic pressure should compensate, while new plasma protein is produced. The amount of blood and crystalloid required should be dictated by maintenance of hematocrit over 30%, with adequate restoration of central venous pressure, vital signs, and urine flow. In patients with evidence of heart disease the monitoring of these parameters requires very particular care to guard against the development of congestive heart failure.

The use of colloid solutions such as plasma or albumin has come under increasing criticism for several reasons. First, there is risk of hepatitis from plasma. Second, plasma, water, and electrolytes equilibrate with the ECF rapidly, leaving the albumin in the intravascular compartment, and albumin is rapidly metabolized (34). Third, the infusion of solutions containing albumin may contribute to pulmonary dysfunction, since there may be increased pulmonary capillary permeability to albumin in shock (35). Finally, these solutions are expensive. These considerations, as well as lack of clear-cut evidence to show superiority of colloids over crystalloids in the treatment of hemorrhagic shock, would indicate that colloid therapy has a limited place in the resuscitation of the patient with gastrointestinal blood loss, unless severe hypoalbuminemia persists, such as in the cirrhotic patient.

Drugs

The use of vasoconstrictive agents in early hemorrhagic shock has been largely abandoned because of the better understanding of the systemic responses to hemorrhage. Vasoconstriction is maximal under these conditions, and the addition of exogenous vasoconstrictors not only fails to correct the underlying problems of hypovolemia, but may prevent adequate volume replacement by elevation of the blood pressure. Furthermore, the additional risk of cardiac arrhythmias, as well as experimental evidence showing increased mortality with the use of vasoconstrictors (36), would justify the condemnation of the use of these agents in the initial treatment of hemorrhagic shock.

The use of vasodilators, initially recommended by Wiggers (37), to improve tissue perfusion by reversal of vasoconstriction, remains controversial. Experimental and clinical data have been contradictory (38). Shoemaker and Brown, in their clinical study (38), concluded that the addition of vasodilators to volume therapy was beneficial only because the former permitted adequate replacement of volume due to the increased fluid space provided by vasodilatation.

LATE SHOCK

Untreated, prolonged hemorrhagic shock will result in anoxic cellular damage that will ultimately give rise to progressive organ failure, culminating in ventricular dysfunction and death. Clinically, the later stages of shock are heralded by persistent hypotension, lactic acidemia, metabolic acidosis, and oliguria despite adequate volume replacement. Edema, under these circumstances is not unusual, reflecting increased capillary permeability with extravasation of administered fluids into the tissues. It is this stage of shock that has often been called "irreversible," but the choice of the term is unfortunate because it implies that further resuscitative measures will fail. If, however, it is acknowledged that body organs have a great capacity to regain normal function despite extensive cell damage, then resuscitative efforts should never cease until all therapeutic measures have been exhausted, and the patient has been pronounced dead.

The treatment of late and profound shock necessitates the use of more accurate measurements of the cardiovascular status. Under these circumstances, central venous pressure (CVP), pulmonary artery pressure, and pulmonary wedge pressure measurements are invaluable in dictating therapy. The CVP line is easily inserted and can be extremely valuable as a guide to fluid management provided that its limitations are realized. The CVP levels are extremely sensitive to changes in intrathoracic pressure and, hence, are readily affected by respiratory movements, positive end-expiratory pressure, and intrathoracic pathology such as pneumo- or hemothorax. Furthermore, the central veins, the right heart, and pulmonary veins are extremely distensible, and rapid volume changes may not, therefore, be reflected by appropriate changes in CVP levels. Despite these limitations, the CVP is a useful adjunct in the management of the patient in shock when serial measurements are recorded to observe the trends of response to therapy. However, because of the above considerations, the Swan-Ganz catheter has gained increasing use in recent years (39). This catheter is easily directed into the pulmonary artery via an antecubital vein and, with its balloon inflated into the "wedged" position, it can measure left atrial pressure. Furthermore, cardiac output can be measured by the Fick principle using this catheter. It should be recognized, however, that left atrial pressure measurements with the Swan-Ganz catheter can be affected by high levels of positive end-expiratory pressure where pulmonary capillary pressure is exceeded by alveolar pressure. Nevertheless, because of the much lower compliance of the pulmonary venous circuit and left heart, the Swan-Ganz catheter is a much more sensitive device for monitoring changes in the cardiovascular status of the patient, than is the CVP line. It does, however, require appropriate recording equipment and trained personnel for its use. Placement of intraarterial catheters is also helpful in monitoring of blood pressure and arterial blood gases.

Since the treatment of late shock is difficult and has limited success, every effort must be made to prevent its development by early aggressive management of the volume-depleted patient, as we have already discussed. When volume and oxygen carrying capacity have been restored as judged by the parameters just discussed and yet shock persists with increasing evidence of ventricular dysfunction, then other therapeutic measures must be instituted as guided by frequent assessments of cardiovascular function.

1. *Dopamine.* This sympathomimetic drug has gained increasing use in recent years. This drug improves cardiac output by stimulation of B-adrenergic receptors (40), while it has a fairly low toxicity in that production of cardiac arrhythmias is infrequent. Tachyphylaxis is rare. Additionally, dopamine improves renal blood flow and can reverse incipient renal failure. Dosage can be titrated depending on blood pressure and CVP or pulmonary wedge pressures.

2. *Isoproterenol.* This drug is an effective inotropic and chronotropic agent. Its use in late hemorrhagic shock, however, is limited because of its potential in the production of severe cardiac arrhythmias, much more so than dopamine. It may be used, however, in the less frequent situations where the heart rate is slow while cardiac output is depressed in late shock.

3. *Digitalis.* If pulmonary wedge pressures and CVP are high and hypotension persists, then digitalis administration should be considered. Frequently, the improvement in left ventricular function will reverse the falling tissue perfusion under these circumstances, while tissue oxygenation will be improved if hypoxia due to pulmonary edema is present.

4. *Mannitol.* This agent may well become a mainstay in the treatment of late shock. It can rapidly increase the intravascular and extracellular fluid compartments by its osmotic effects. Its usefulness in prevention of acute renal failure is well documented (41). Furthermore, it has been shown to be effective in reduction of brain and lung edema (42,43). It may also improve coronary blood flow (44). Mannitol may be of extreme value in the clinical situation of late shock when, after fluid resuscitation, persistent hypotension and massive edema are present. Under these circumstances, mannitol will reduce intracellular as well as interstitial edema, and thus improve nutrient supply to the cells. Its administration must be monitored carefully to prevent cardiac failure. Judicious combination with loop diuretics and cardiac inotropic agents will prevent cardiac decompensation in this setting. Constant drip infusion of mannitol in the above situations is now under investigation.

5. *Steroids.* The use of massive doses of adrenocortico steroids in shock is a subject of much controversy and heated debate. The rationale for their use has been based on experimental observations that they may stabilize lysosomal and cell mem-

branes, thereby improving metabolic function and reversing deterioration of the cardiovascular system (45). The benefits in the clinical situation have been difficult to document, and over the years there has developed a dictum that "no patient should be allowed to die in shock without a trial of steroids." This not only lacks scientific merit, but without careful documentation to the contrary, may be harmful in the treatment of late shock.

Renal Support in Hemorrhagic Shock (Scheme 4-3)

Adequate volume replacement is the mainstay in prevention of renal failure in hemorrhagic shock. Careful monitoring of urine output is crucial. Daily measurements of creatinine clearance (a 1-hr collection is sufficient), osmolarity, and sodium concentration are invaluable for the recognition of incipient renal failure. Oliguria, falling creatinine clearance, rising sodium concentration (> 60 mEq/liter) are the warning signs. Urine osmolarity approaches that of the plasma in incipient renal failure. Urine : plasma creatinine ratios above 20 indicate continued volume depletion, while ratios below 15 indicate acute tubular necrosis. Another sensitive test for recognition of early renal failure is the calculation of free water clearance (46), since free water retention is a prelude to acute renal failure.

If volume replacement has been thought to be adequate, and yet some of the above findings indicating incipient renal failure are present, a CVP (and if available, a pulmonary artery catheter) should be inserted to assess cardiovascular status. Low CVP or pulmonary artery and wedge pressure would indicate the need for further volume restoration. A rapid infusion of isosmotic crystalloid or 25 grams of mannitol will quickly establish reversibility of incipient renal failure if diuresis is the result. Under these circumstances, continued vigorous fluid therapy will correct oliguria as volume is restored.

On the contrary, if the CVP or pulmonary arterial and wedge pressures are high in the presence of incipient renal failure, then loop diuretics should be given, in combination with cardiac inotropic agents if indicated. The use of massive doses of loop diuretics have been advocated in this situation because these agents can

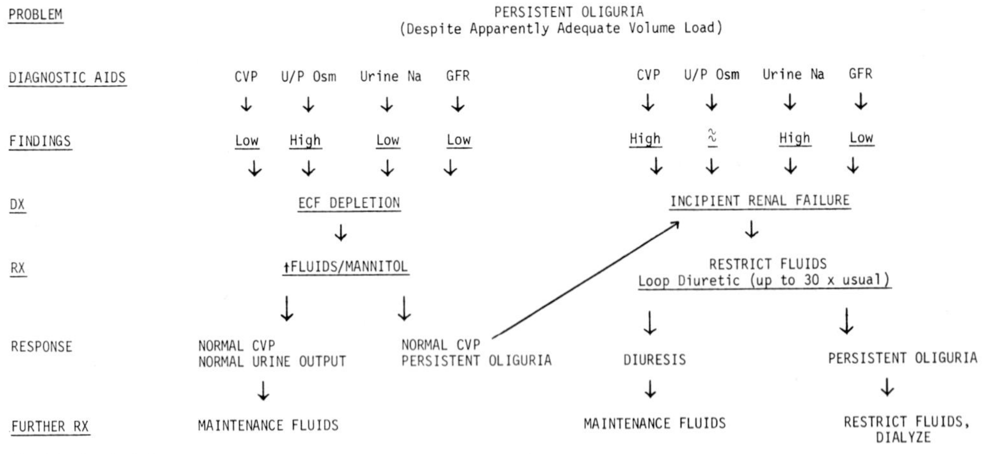

SCHEME 4-3

theoretically reverse the marked cortical vasoconstriction (47). Recently, this concept has been challenged by Epstein et al, who suggest, that without full substantiation of the claims of others, these large doses of diuretics may be more harmful than beneficial (48). Despite this controversy, the short-term use of large doses of loop diuretics may well be effective in preventing acute renal failure in selected patients, in whom volume replacement has been adequate and who show evidence of early, reversible renal failure.

REFERENCES

1. Moore, F. D.: *Metabolic Care of the Surgical Patient.* W. B. Saunders Co., Philadelphia, 1960.
2. Wiggers, C. J.: *Physiology of Shock.* The Commonwealth Fund, New York, 1950.
3. Shires, G. T., Carrico, C. J., Canizaco, P. C.: Shock: in *Major Problems in Surgery*, Vol. XIII. W. B. Saunders Co., Philadelphia, 1973.
4. Farrell, G. L.: Physiological factors which influence secretion of aldosterone. *Recent Progr. Hormone Res.* **15:**275, 1959.
5. Coswell, J. W., Guyton, A. C.: Further evidence favoring a cardiac mechanism in irreversible hemmorrhagic shock. *Amer. J. Physiol.* **203:**248, 1962.
6. Baue, A. E., Wirth, M. A., and Sayeed, M. M.: The dynamics of altered ATP dependent and ATP yielding cell processes in shock. *Surgery,* **72:**94, 1972.
7. Schumer, W.: Localization of the energy pathway block in shock. *Surgery,* **64:**55, 1968.
8. Shires, T., Cunningham, J. N., Baher, C. R. F., Reeder, S. F., Illner, H., Wagner, I. Y., and Maher, J.: Alterations in cellular membrane function during hemorrhagic shock in primates. *Ann. Surg.* **176:**288, 1972.
9. Prutenburg, A. M., Bell, M. L., and Butcher, R. W. et al: Adenosine 3'5' monophosphate levels in hemorrhagic shock. *Ann. Surg.* **174:**461, 1971.
10. Lillehei, R. C., and Dietzman, R. H.: Circulatory collapse and shock, in *Principles of Surgery*, 2nd Ed., McGraw-Hill, New York, 1974.
11. Jones, R. C., and Wangensteen, S. L.: Protective influence of cathepsin D antiserum in hemorrhagic shock. *Surg. Forum,* **XXVI:**29, 1975.
12. Cloutier, C. T., Lowery, B. D., and Carey, L. C.: Acid-base disturbances in hemorrhagic shock. *Arch. Surg.* **98:**551, 1969.
13. Schumer, W., and Kukral, J. C.: Metabolism of shock. *Surgery,* **63:**630, 1968.
14. Vladeck. B. C., Bassin, R., Kark, A. E., and Shoemaker, W. C.: Rapid and slow hemorrhage in man: II. Sequential acid-base and oxygen transport responses. *Ann. Surg.* **173:**331, 1971.
15. Carey, L. C., Lowery, B. D., and Cloutier, C. T.: Hemorrhagic shock. *Current Probl. Surg.* 1971.
16. Benesch, R., and Benesch, R. E.: The effect of organic phosphates from the human erythrocyte on the allosteric properties of hemoglobin. *Biochim. Biophys. Res. Commun.* **26:**162, 1967.

17. Moss, G. S., and Saletta, J. D.: Current Concepts: Traumatic shock in man. *New Engl. J. Med.* **290:**724, 1974.

18. Ryan, N. T., George, B. C., Egdahl, D. H., and Egdahl, R. H.: Chronic tissue insulin resistance following hemorrhagic shock. *Ann. Surg.* **180:**402, 1974.

19. McNamara, J. J., Molot, M. D., Dunn, R. A. et al: Effect of hypertonic glucose in hypovolemic shock in man. *Ann. Surg.* **176:**247, 1973.

20. Chaudry, I. H., Sayeed, M. M., and Baue, A.E.: Reversal of insulin resistance by in vivo infusion of ATP in experimental shock. *Surg. Forum,* **XXVI:**44, 1975.

21. Skinner, S. L., McGubbin, J. W., Page, I. H.: Control of renin secretion. *Circ. Res.* **15:**64, 1964.

22. Schumer, W., and Nyhus, L. M.: *Treatment of shock.* Lea and Febiger, Philadelphia, 1974.

23. Moore, F. D., Lyons, J., Pierce, E. C., Morgan, A. P., Drinker, P. A., MacArthur, J. D., and Dammin, G. J.: *Post-traumatic pulmonary insufficiency.* W. B. Saunders, Philadelphia, 1969.

24. Buckberg, G. D., Lipman, C. A., Hahn, J. A., Smith, M. J., and Hennessey, J. A.: Pulmonary changes following hemorrhagic shock and resuscitation in baboons. *J. Thorac. Cardiovasc. Surg.* **59:**450, 1970.

25. Moss, G. S., DasGupta, T. K., Newson, B. et al: Effect of hemorrhagic shock on pulmonary interstitial sodium distribution in the primate lung. *Ann. Surg.* **177:**211, 1973.

26. Garvey, J. W., Hagstrom, J. W., and Veith, F. J.: Pathologic pulmonary changes in hemorrhagic shock. *Ann. Surg.* **181:**870, 1975.

27. McClelland, R. N., Shires, G. T., Banter, C. R., Coln, C. D., and Carrico, J.: Balanced salt solution in the treatment of hemorrhagic shock. *JAMA,* **199:**930, 1967.

28. Prentice, T., Olney, J. M., Artz, C. P., and Howard, J. M.: Studies of blood volume and transfusion therapy in the Korean battle casualties. *Surg. Gyn. Obstet.* **99:**542, 1954.

29. Miller, P. P., Robbins, T. O., Tong, M. J. et al: Coagulation defects associated with massive blood transfusions. *Ann. Surg.* **174:**794, 1971.

30. Boyan, C. P., Howland, W.S.: Blood temperature: A critical factor in massive transfusion. *Anesthesiol.* **22:**559, 1961.

31. Bentler, E., Meul, A., and L. A. Wood: Depletion and regeneration of 2,3-diphosphoglyceric acid in stored red blood cells. *Transfusion,* **9:**109, 1969.

32. Valen, C. R.: Viability and function of preserved red cells. *New Engl. J. Med.* **284:**81, 1971.

33. Dillon, J., Lynch, L. J., Meyers, R., Butcher, H. R., and Moyer, C. A.: A bioassay of treatment of hemorrhagic shock. *Arch. Surg.* **93:**537, 1966.

34. Moore, F. D.: The effects of hemorrhage on body composition. *New Engl. J. Med.* **273:**567, 1965.

35. Siegel, D. C., Moss, G. S., and Cochin, A.: Pulmonary changes following treatment of hemorrhagic shock: Saline versus colloid infusion. *Surg. Forum,* **21:**17, 1970.

36. Close, S. A. et al: The effect of norepinephrine on survival in experimental acute hypotension. *Surg. Forum,* **8:**22, 1957.

37. Wiggers, H. C. et al: Vasoconstriction and the development of irreversible hemorrhagic shock. *Am. J. Physiol.* **153:**511, 1948.

38. Shoemaker, W. C., and Brown, R. S.: The dilemma of vasopressors and vasodilators in treatment of shock. *Surg. Gyn. Obstet.* **132:**51, 1971.
39. Swan, H. J. C., Ganz, W., Forrester, J., Marcus, H., Diamond, G., and Chonette, D.: Catheterization of the heart in man with use of a flow-directed balloon-tipped catheter. *New Engl. J. Med.* **283:**447, 1970.
40. Loeb, H. S., Winslow, E.B., and Rohimtoola, S. A.: Acute hemodynamic effects of dopamine in patients with shock. *Circulation,* **44:**163, 1971.
41. Powers, S. R., Boba, A., Hostnik, W., and Stein, A.: Prevention of post-operative acute renal failure with mannitol in 100 cases. *Surgery,* **55:**15, 1964.
42. Wise, B. L., and Carter, N.: The value of hypertonic mannitol solution in decreasing brain mass and lowering cerebrospinal fluid pressure. *J. Neurosurg.* **19:**1058, 1963.
43. Williams, O. D., Ozznert, K., and Boggett, R. W.: Hyperosmolar perfusion for removal of pulmonary edema. *J. Surg. Res.* **12:**105, 1972.
44. Williams, J. T., Curry, G. C., Atkins, J. M., Parkey, R. and Harwitz, L. R.: Influence of hypertonic mannitol on ventricular performance and coronary blood flow in patients. *Circulation,* **51:**1095, 1975.
45. Schumer, W., and Nyhus, L. M.: Corticosteroid effect on biochemical parameters of human oligenic shock. *Arch. Surg.* **100:**405, 1970.
46. Baek, S. M., Brown, R. S., and Shoemaker, W. C.: Early prediction of acute renal failure with free water clearance. *Surg. Forum,* **23:**79, 1972.
47. Birtch, A. G., Zakheim, R. M., Jones, L. G., and Bargen, A. C.: Redistribution of renal blood flow produced by furosamide and ethacrynic acid. *Circ. Res.* **21:**869, 1967.
48. Epstein, M., Schneider, N. S., and Befeler, B.: Effect of intrarenal furosamide on renal function and intrarenal hemodynamics on renal function in acute renal failure. *Am. J. Med.* **58:**510, 1975.

5

MANAGEMENT

In the preceding chapters the clinical presentation, initial evaluation, and provisional diagnosis of the patient with gastrointestinal bleeding is reviewed. We also discuss the methods for confirming the clinical diagnosis by means of endoscopy and selective arteriography. The physiologic basic for restoring the circulatory status of patients with massive blood loss, which is a prerequisite for their proper management, is treated in detail.

In this chapter we consider:

1. Medical management, including a discussion of the general principles applicable to all patients with bleeding from the gastrointestinal tract, as well as the special points applicable to individual disease states.
2. The appropriate timing of barium contrast studies.
3. The indications for the use of intraarterial infusion of vasoconstrictor agents.
4. The indications for surgical intervention.
5. The selection of appropriate surgical procedures.

In the case of patients with occult bleeding, no urgent decision needs to be made. The problem is one of making a definitive diagnosis, and on that basis deciding whether continued conservative therapy or an elective surgical procedure will best serve the long-term interests of the patient. On the other hand, in the case of patients with overt gastrointestinal bleeding the decision must be made between continued medical treatment, a continued medical program with subsequent elective surgical treatment, or emergency surgical intervention. The major factors that must be considered in arriving at the right decision in any individual include an estimate of the magnitude of blood loss, the nature of the bleeding lesion, the age of the patient, and the presence of complicating intercurrent disease.

ESTIMATE OF BLOOD LOSS

Determination of the magnitude of blood loss is often difficult. The history as given by the patient or the relatives is often quite "inaccurate" as an estimate of volume lost. The amount of blood lost may be minimized out of fear, or exaggerated because of dilution in the water of the toilet bowl. The pulse rate and blood pressure are helpful especially if what is normal for that particular patient is known. Unfortunately, this is rarely the case. Tibbs, based on a study of 33 patients, found that although an elevation of pulse rate and fall in blood pressure were helpful as a rough guide, their correlation with blood volume measured by Evans blue dye was poor (1). The degree of peripheral pallor was a fairly good guide to peripheral vasoconstriction and thus to volume loss in Tibbs' experience (1). Tudhope (2), however, was unable to confirm this finding. Using Cr^{51} labeled autologous red blood cells, Tudhope showed an excellent correlation between red cell mass and hemoglobin 24 hours after hemorrhage, but not before that time (2). Hence, this observation is consistent with previous findings by Evert, Stead, and Gibson in 1941 (3), who demonstrated that following a 1000-ml phlebotomy only about 30% of circulatory volume was restored in 2 hours, while 50% was restored by 8 hours. Tudhope (2) found that patients with a systolic blood pressure below 100 mm Hg always had a much reduced red cell mass. But a higher systolic presure did not rule out major volume depletion. Similarly a pulse rate above 110 per minute correlated well with a reduced cell mass. Lack of tachycardia was not, however, evidence against significant blood loss. A hemoglobin of less than 12 gm per 100 ml on admission in previously healthy subjects indicated that more than 50% of red cell mass had been lost (2). In this study of 30 patients, 17 were found to have lost 50% or more of their red cell mass. These observations show that while vital signs, skin turgor, and peripheral pallor can give an indication of the magnitude of blood loss, the correlation of abnormalities in these clinical signs with severe volume depletion is only a rough one. Continued complaint of thirst, especially in a restless patient, even in the absence of hypotension or tachycardia, is strong additional evidence of volume depletion.

Therefore, other evidence must be sought to help establish the extent of volume depletion. As already indicated, the hematocrit is not a good indicator of the magnitude of initial blood loss less than 24 hours after an acute hemorrhage. As we discuss in Chapter 4, however, it may be a good guide as to the immediate requirement for red cell transfusion, with values below 30% indicating the need for such therapy. This may indicate preexisting anemia, presumably due to chronic blood loss. A urine output of less than 30 ml per hr implies loss of more than 30% of extracellular fluid, and consequent renal hypoperfusion. Under these circumstances, urinary sodium excretion is likely to be low (< 20 mEq/liter). The measurement of central venous pressure is the most readily available method for determining the adequacy of intravascular volume. However, in patients with cardiac or pulmonary disease the central venous pressure as measured by a line in the superior vena cava may be misleading. For example, it may be in the apparently normal range (8 to 14 cm H_2O) because of coexisting right heart failure, which will tend to raise the pressure, and dehydration, which will tend to lower it. In these patients accurate measurement requires determination of wedged pulmonary artery pressure by using a Swan-Ganz catheter and a pressure recorder as described in Chapter 4. Nevertheless, a central venous pressure catheter may still yield valuable information, when the more elaborate methods are not available. Furthermore, monitoring of the central venous pressure is a most helpful guide to proper fluid replacement, since restoration of a low CVP to normal, especially if urine volume rises, is a good indication of adequate fluid replacement. On the other hand, a rise in CVP appreciably above normal values indicates either fluid overload or incipient cardiac decompensation.

Patients with evidence of major gastrointestinal hemorrhage should be admitted to a service with special experience in the management of those patients if such a service is available. These units may be primarily medical (4), or surgical (5), and they function best when run in close cooperation between the medical and surgical teams, with the help of experienced nursing staff. The latter is most important, since careful clinical monitoring of the patient is the best way to determine whether bleeding has stopped, is continuing, or has recurred.

MONITORING OF THE PATIENT

The critical time for recurrence of bleeding, at least in patients with upper gastrointestinal hemorrhage, is during the first 36 hours after admission to the hospital (6). This is also a period during which the patient's condition is most likely to be unstable. Therefore, it is during the first 2 days that the patient will need the most intensive observation. The patient's pulse and blood pressure, and urine output should be recorded hourly. The presence of thirst and agitation must be noted as well as complaints of continued abdominal pain (Table 5-1). Some have felt that in patients with upper gastrointestinal bleeding, a nasogastric tube should be kept in place as a way of detecting continuing or recurrent bleeding. However, there is a lack of good data to support this contention. For example, Dawson, in a study of 100 consecutive patients with upper gastrointestinal bleeding, found that rebleeding was diagnosed by clinical signs in all but one patient, although a nasogastric tube was used in all patients (7). On the other hand, Chandler and Watkinson (8) in a similar series reported that frequent gastric aspirations were helpful in the early detection of recurrent hemorrhage. Since the evidence for the value of gastric aspirations in detecting recurrent bleeding is unconvincing, we prefer to remove nasogastric tubes once the presence or absence of blood in the stomach has been established, since this is most comfortable for the patient. However, if the facilities for monitoring the patient are limited, a nasogastric tube may well yield valuable information in patients with upper gastrointestinal bleeding.

Once the patient has been admitted to the unit the aim of therapy is to ensure adequate volume and red cell replacement. Persisting thirst, agitation, or anxiety despite sedation, tachycardia, and hypotension indicate that *volume replacement* has been *inadequate.* As indicated in Table 5-1, this may be due to *continuing blood loss* or insufficient replacement therapy. In both instances, urine output will be low (< 30 cc/hr). In patients who are continuing to bleed, bowel sounds are usually hyperactive, with frequent bloody or tarry stools. In contrast, bowel sounds will usually be normal or hypoactive in patients who have stopped bleeding. The continued presence of occult blood in the stool does not necessarily indicate continuing hemorrhage. Schiff and colleagues (16) demonstrated that occult blood may be present for three days after instillation of as little as 125 ml of blood into the stomach, and for 5 to 12 days after gastric administration of 1000 to 2000 ml of blood. Indeed, in the latter case, melena was noted for 1 to 5 days. Since the hematocrit does not equilibrate for 24 to 36 hours after an acute bleeding episode, it may be a poor guide to continuing hemorrhage, although as mentioned previously a value below 30% may be an indication for blood transfusion. A rising hematocrit, if associated with tachycardia, hypotension, or thirst, is an indication of continuing volume depletion. It is only when the hematocrit becomes stable or actually rises, while pulse rate and

Table 5-1
Monitoring the Patient

Observation	Interpretation	Further Evidence	Action
1. Persistent tachycardia and hypotension	a. Inadequate volume replacement	Urine volume low, thrist, bowel sounds OK	Increased electrolyte, fluid and blood replacement
	b. Continued bleeding	Active bowel sounds, blood in stool or stomach	As above + surgery/pitressin
2. Continued agitation and thirst	a. Continued bleeding	Active bowel sounds Blood in stool or stomach	As above
	b. Bowel infarction	Absent bowel sounds Blood in stool	Laparotomy
3. Fall in BP, rise in pulse rate and/or recurrence of thirst and anxiety	Recurrence of bleeding	Recurrence of thirst Blood in stool Blood in stomach	Fluid and blood replacement Surgery/pitressin
4. Persistent oliguria*	a. Inadequate volume replacement	CVP $\downarrow$ Urine Na$^+$ $\downarrow$ Urine osmols $\uparrow$	Increased fluid replacement
	b. Acute tubular necrosis	CVP—variable Urine Na$^+$ $\uparrow$ Urine isotonic	If CVP $\downarrow$ try fluid challenge Otherwise restrict fluids
5. Persistent abdominal pain	a. Penetrating ulcer	UGI bleed Ulcer demonstrated	Early surgery
	b. Inflammatory lesion	Lower GI bleed Abdominal mass	Antibiotics? Early surgery?
	c. Bowel infarction	Silent abdomen	$\Big\{$ Immediate surgery
	d. Perforation	Free air	

*The problem of persistent oliguria is discussed fully in Chapter 4.

blood pressure return to normal, that it indicates adequate replacement therapy. At this point the CVP should have returned to normal (10-14 cm saline) and urine output to 50 ml per hr or greater. Failure to attain this state should suggest continuing blood loss. Alternatively, the possibility of some acute intraabdominal complication, such as bowel infarction or perforation should also be considered. In these two situations, bowel sounds will be absent and signs of acute peritoneal irritation will be present. This latter situation requires immediate massive volume replacement and surgical intervention. In the former situation the decision will be between selective angiography and vasopressin infusion and surgical therapy. This decision will be discussed later in this chapter.

Recurrence of bleeding is generally regarded as an indication for surgical intervention, since it is associated with a steeply rising mortality with continued conservative therapy (4,9). Recurrence of bleeding should be suspected when a patient, whose vital signs have been stabilized, again complains of abdominal discomfort and thirst, becomes anxious, and has a fall in blood pressure, rise in pulse rate, and active bowel sounds (Table 5-1). In patients with upper gastrointestinal bleeding a gastric aspirate may confirm the clinical impression of recurrent hemorrhage. Reappearance of fresh blood in bowel movements will confirm the presence of lower gastrointestinal bleeding. Thus the diagnosis of major recurrent hemorrhage can be made readily on clinical grounds. Lesser degrees of renewed bleeding are more difficult to detect. In this situation, reliance must be placed on a falling hematocrit and the reappearance of occult blood in the stool. Since the measurement of the hematocrit is not precise, a decrease in this determination must be confirmed by repeated measurement.

Persistent oliguria may indicate either inadequate volume replacement or acute tubular necrosis (Table 5-1). The differential diagnosis of these two situations is very important, since their proper management is quite different. This problem has been reviewed in more detail in Chapter 4. If volume replacement has been inadequate, renal perfusion will be diminished. In this situation, intrinsic renal function is well preserved and, therefore, renal conservation of sodium and of free water will be maximal, resulting in a hyperosmolar urine with low sodium content ($<$ 10 mEq/liter). The CVP will be low in such patients ($<$ 10 cm saline). By contrast in the patient with acute tubular necrosis, due to prolonged hypovolemia and hypotension, urinary sodium excretion is high and the urine is isotonic with plasma. The patient with persistent hypovolemia clearly will need increased fluid replacement with isotonic electrolyte solution. It is helpful in such patients to monitor the CVP and to continue vigorous intravenous fluid administration until the CVP returns to normal levels, when urine output should rise. If under these circumstances, oliguria persists, an attempt should be made to induce diuresis by means of an osmotic load, such as 20% mannitol, or with the use of a loop diuretic, such as furosamide. In patients who require such drastic measures, an indwelling urethral catheter should be placed so that urine flow can be readily measured. A CVP line is also necessary in such patients to permit constant monitoring of circulating volume. The patient with evidence of intrinsic renal failure (ATN) must be given intravenous fluids with great care, since fluid overload in patients of this kind is extremely difficult to correct. If the CVP is low, fluids may be given, while urine output is carefully recorded, until the CVP rises to normal. If urine flow does not improve, an osmotic load or preferably a loop diuretic may be tried. If this fails to induce diuresis, fluid replacement must be restricted to replacement of measured losses plus 500 ml to make up for insensible losses. This latter volume may be increased if significant fever is present. Once the diagnosis of ATN is suspected, consultation with a nephrologist is advisable.

Persistent abdominal pain (Table 5-1) in a patient with bleeding must be regarded as a serious problem, since it may indicate the need for urgent surgical intervention. In a patient with a proved peptic ulcer, continuing pain despite proper therapy for ulcer disease may indicate impending or actual perforation, or penetration of the ulcer. Absence of bowel sounds, especially when associated with a finding of a rigid abdomen, or other signs of peritoneal irritation in such a patient strongly suggests perforation and should prompt immediate radiologic examination of the abdomen to look for free air, and if confirmed, should lead to surgical treatment. Continuing bleeding in the face of a silent or rigid abdomen suggests bowel infarction and is an absolute indication for immediate laparotomy. In the patient with lower intestinal bleeding and persisting pain, especially if a palpable tender mass is present, a localized inflammatory process such as a pericolic abscess must be considered. Such patients need surgical management as a general rule.

OTHER GENERAL CONSIDERATIONS

Hemorrhage from the digestive tract naturally causes the patient considerable anxiety. Therefore, one of the main aims of therapy should be to *relieve anxiety*. The patient must, therefore, be given appropriate sedation. In patients free of liver and lung disease, this may be accomplished by use of barbiturates or morphine. No good data exist to show that adequate sedation helps to arrest bleeding; however, it is the general consensus that sedation is beneficial in relieving the patient's anxiety. Caution must be used in the administration of sedatives to patients with pulmonary insufficiency. In these patients, respiratory depressants, such as barbiturates and morphine, should be avoided. Diazepam used with care is a useful agent in such patients. Patients with liver disease, alcoholic or posthepatitic, are another group in whom the use of sedative drugs presents a special problem. Most of the generally used sedatives require hepatic metabolism, and this is predictably impaired in such patients (10,11). Morphine and codeine should not be used in these patients. The short-acting barbiturates, such as phenobarbital, which have significant renal excretion, are relatively safe, if used with care. Diazepam may also be used with caution.

Another group of patients who present a particularly difficult problem are those who have been imbibing large amounts of ethanol (12). Two kinds of problems are encountered in this group of patients, namely an excessive drug affect in patients who ingested alcohol within a few hours of admission, or greatly increased drug tolerance in chronic alcoholics, who have not taken ethanol in the 12 to 24 hours prior to admission. Ethanol is in part metabolized by the same microsomal enzyme system responsible for oxidation of many drugs (12). In patients who have recently ingested ethanol, this enzyme system may be fully occupied with ethanol oxidation, and not available for drug metabolism. Therefore, in such patients a normal dose of a sedative drug, such as a barbiturate, may have a much exaggerated effect and could prove fatal. Conversely, since the microsomal drug metabolizing enzyme system is induceable by ethanol, a chronic alcoholic, without severe liver damage, may metabolize a sedative agent very rapidly, and thus require much larger doses than normally needed for a sedative effect. Therefore, in patients known to ingest large amounts of alcoholic beverages, an attempt should be made to determine when they last did so, and to adjust the dose of medication accordingly. Furthermore, these patients should be kept under particularly careful observation.

The problem of elucidating disorders of the clotting system have already been reviewed in Chapter 2. All patients with gastrointestinal bleeding should have had at least a prothrombin time determination as part of their initial evaluation. If possible, a platelet count and an activated partial thromboplastin time (APTT) should also have been obtained. If these are normal, no special treatment is indicated; however, it is generally recommended, and we agree, that after each 4 to 5 units of packed red cells or of whole bank blood, a unit of fresh frozen plasma should be given to restore clotting factors absent in bank blood (see Chapter 4). When abnormalities of clotting function are demonstrated, appropriate replacement therapy must be undertaken. If time permits a full evaluation with factor assays may be helpful in planning therapy. If the platelet count and bleeding time are normal, but the prothrombin time is prolonged, parenteral vitamin K should be tried. If the APTT is also prolonged, or if it is prolonged in the face of a normal PT (Table 2-4), fresh frozen plasma will be needed for correction. In this situation a hematologic consultation should be obtained, since the management of the patient will be greatly aided by complete elucidation of the nature of the coagulation defect.

INDICATION FOR SURGICAL INTERVENTION

The precise indications for *emergency surgery* in patients with gastrointestinal bleeding will vary depending on the precise diagnosis and will be discussed further in the context of the major diagnostic categories. However, there are some general principles that apply in all cases. Potentially all patients whose bleeding fails to stop within 12 hours of admission to the hospital or whose bleeding recurs after admission must be considered candidates for emergency surgical treatment. This is especially true of patients over the age of 50, and who have a history of one or more prior bleeding episodes. Suspected complications such as perforation, infarction of bowel, or abscess formation are additional reasons for emergency surgery.

These indications must, however, be evaluated individually in the light of the general condition of the particular patient. Thus for example, a recent myocardial infarction (< 4 to 6 weeks earlier) is generally regarded as a contraindication to anesthesia and surgical intervention, because of the unstable state of the myocardium and the threat of ventricular fibrillation. However, in a patient with a chronic peptic ulcer, the risks of continued or repeated massive hemorrhage, with consequent myocardial hypoperfusion, may represent a higher risk than that of an operation. Other intercurrent illnesses, such as pneumonia, may also raise problems. In general, we believe the patient's interests are best served by close consultation between a surgically minded internist and a conservative surgeon, as so aptly stated by Avery Jones (13). The availability of intraarterial selective pitressin infusion now provides a possible alternative to surgery in some high-risk patients. The proper role of this form of therapy has not yet been fully established, but will be reviewed later in this chapter.

The indications for *elective surgery* are more strongly influenced by the specific diagnosis, the magnitude of blood loss, and whether this is a first episode of hemorrhage or one of several recurrences. This problem will, therefore, be reviewed under the specific diagnostic categories.

FEEDING THE PATIENT

There is still no general agreement on whether patients with overt gastrointestinal bleeding should be fed or fasted in the first 24 to 48 hours after admission. Some authorities feel that, since in patients with upper gastrointestinal hemorrhage recurrence of bleeding is most likely in the first 36 hours, food should be withheld during this period and nasogastric suction continued. We have already indicated that there is little data to support the value of continued nasogastric suction for the early detection of recurrent bleeding. Furthermore, should surgery become necessary, milk and liquid antacids can readily be removed from the stomach with a large bore tube, while the patient and the operating room are readied. We, therefore, advocate feeding patients with upper gastrointestinal bleeding with milk plus antacids, if they are able to tolerate this. After 36 to 48 hours the patient, if stable, can then be advanced to a bland diet with antacids after and between meals. The problem is different in patients with bleeding esophageal varices. Such patients may have to be placed on a protein restricted diet (see below). In such patients, antacids with oral fluids containing carbohydrates are appropriate.

In patients with lower intestinal bleeding, emergency surgery is relatively rarely necessary. They may, however, benefit from bowel rest. Such patients should, therefore, be offered a low residue, low roughage diet. This can be accomplished by use of clear liquids or one of the newer formula feedings.

SPECIFIC DISEASE STATES

Upper gastrointestinal bleeding (See Schemes 2-1 and 2-2)

Peptic ulcer disease.   Gastric and duodenal ulcer between them account for 40% to 50% of all causes of upper gastrointestinal bleeding (Table 2-1, Chapter 2) (9,14). Patients with peptic ulcer are, therefore, the largest single group in this category. The clinical features that suggest a diagnosis of either gastric or duodenal ulcer are briefly reviewed in Chapter 2. The clinical features are often clear-cut and make a diagnosis relatively straightforward, when present. However, it is important to bear in mind that 38% of patients with a previously established diagnosis of duodenal ulcer, and 67% of those with gastric ulcer, were found by Palmer to be bleeding from a site other than the previously diagnosed ulcer (14). Furthermore, in many instances the actual bleeding site itself was not radiologically demonstrable. These observations make a most potent argument in favor of early gastrointestinal panendoscopy in the investigation of patients with hemorrhage of the upper digestive tract. These considerations are fully reviewed in Chapters 2 and 3. As indicated, we believe that a precise diagnosis will assist the physician in planning the management of the patient. This view is endorsed by two recent reports. In a study of 208 patients, Cotton et al (14) using an aggressive diagnostic approach obtained an overall mortality rate of 3.8%. This compares with a mortality of 9% reported by Schiller et al (9), also from England, in a larger series of patients in whom endoscopy was rarely used. In Cotton's series 26.4% required emergency surgery (14) compared with 19% in Schiller's series (9). Thus the patients in the two series appear to have had similarly severe bleeding. In a Swedish study, Hellers and Imre (5) noted a significant reduction in mortality, transfusion requirement, and of undiagnosed cases with the adoption of an aggressive diagnostic and surgical policy. Since both these studies are based on retrospective comparisons, neither provides an absolute answer as to the value of early endoscopy for the management, as opposed to the diagnosis, of the patient with upper gastrointestinal hemorrhage.

The diagnosis of peptic ulcer as a source of bleeding can be made with a high degree of accuracy (> 90%) on clinical grounds and panendoscopy (14,17). What then is the role of barium contrast studies of the upper gastrointestinal tract in these patients? A barium x-ray examination can demonstrate a lesion in the upper gastrointestinal tract, but it cannot demonstrate whether that lesion is the source of hemorrhage. We, therefore, believe that the standard upper gastrointestinal series has limited usefulness in the patient with hemorrhage. If endoscopy demonstrates a duodenal ulcer as the bleeding site, a radiologic study is not necessary. If a gastric ulcer is seen to be the source of bleeding at endoscopy, subsequent barium x-ray studies can be used as a means of following healing of the ulcer, if surgery is not undertaken. If, however, an experienced endoscopist is not available, it is evident from the experience of others, who have relied on radiologic diagnosis, that in the great majority of patients successful management is possible without panendoscopy (9,18,19).

Once a diagnosis of bleeding from a peptic ulcer has been established, a plan of management should be made by the team responsible for the patient's care. This plan should be clearly stated. Views on the indications for, and timing of, surgical intervention have evolved gradually over the past 50 years. Initially, surgical intervention was regarded as a last resort (20). Later, the pendulum swung to the other extreme with Finsterer (21) advocating immediate surgical therapy for all patients with upper gastrointestinal bleeding. This view was gradually modified to a selective surgical approach as advocated by Avery Jones (13). This policy recommends operative treatment for patients with bleeding peptic ulcer in whom hermorrhage continues or recurs after admission to the hospital. This attitude to patients with bleeding peptic ulcer is now generally accepted, since it has been shown to be based on well substantiated data on risk factors in this group of patients.

Two large series illustrate this point. Schiller et al (9) reported that 78.6% of their 2149 patients bled only once during any one admission. This group of patients, therefore, would not need emergency surgical treatment. On the other hand, these authors found that 11.9% of their patients continued to bleed for 12 to 24 hours after admission, while 3.5% had repeated episodes of hemorrhage (in 6% data were incomplete). Thus emergency surgery was indicated in 15.4% of their patients. In fact, 27% of the patients were treated surgically. These figures are similar to those reported by Avery Jones (13), who noted recurrent or continuing bleeding in 20.5% among 2011 episodes of bleeding in 1764 patients. The major risk factors that increase the mortality rates in patients with bleeding peptic ulcers are shown in Table 5-2. The overall mortality of patients with chronic gastric ulcer is twice as great (9%-16%) as of patients with chronic duodenal ulcers (5.6%-8%),

Table 5-2
Factors Influencing Mortality in Patients with Bleeding Peptic Ulcer (Based on Data from References 9 and 13)

Factor		*Mortality*	*Reference*
A. Type of ulcer		(in percent)	
	Chronic G.U.	16, 9.3	9,13
	Chronic D.U.	8, 5.6	
	Acute ulcers	2.5	
B. Age of patient			
	< 40	2.7	9
	40-59	4.8	
	60-79	13.5	
	> 80	17.9	
C. Age of patient and type of ulcer			
	Chronic G.U. < 60	13.0	13
	> 60	42.9	
	Chronic D.U. < 60	7.0	
	> 60	44.0	
	Acute ulcer < 60	1.7	
	> 60	22.5	
D. Magnitude of bleed			
	Systolic BP		
	> 100 mm Hg	8	9
	80-99 mm Hg	18	
	< 80 mm Hg		
E. Recurrence of bleeding			
	Single	5 1.7	9,13
	Recurrent	10 21.5	
	Continous	30	

while the mortality in patients with bleeding acute ulcers is only 2.5% (Table 5-2,A.). Since gastric ulcer (peak incidence 45-55 years) tends to occur in older patients than duodenal ulcer (peak incidence 35-45 years), the age of the patient may account for some of the difference in mortality rates (Table 5-2,B.). However, these differences still hold true when correction for age is made (Table 5-2,C.).

For all three types of peptic ulcer the death rate increases with increasing age (Table 5-2,C.). In fact, in patients over 60 years of age, age itself is a more important determinant than the type of ulcer. As might be expected, the severity of the blood loss has an important influence on death rates (Table 5-2,D.). In as far as systolic blood pressure reflects volume loss, it can be seen that mortality increases fourfold as blood pressure falls. Item E. in Table 5-2 shows that death rates increase steeply when bleeding either fails to stop or recurs after hospitalization. Of interest is the observation of Lewin and Truelove (22) that a history of previous hemorrhage from a peptic ulcer did not affect the prognosis for the patent in a subsequent bleeding episode. Indeed, as stated above, it is the age of the patient, rather than that of the ulcer which is important. More recently, Northfield (23) has shown in a retrospective study of 472 patients that rebleeding is most likely to occur in the first 48 hours after admission. He further observed that recurrence of hemorrhage was more likely in patients with hematemesis than melena, large initial bleeds, and in those bleeding from chronic gastric ulcers.

These risk factors must always be kept in mind while treating a patient with a bleeding peptic ulcer. The other considerations involved, such as sedation, feeding, monitoring, and early surgical consultation, have already been discussed. Our favored plan of management is outlined below (see Schemes 2-1 and 2-2).

1. Diagnosis is based on history and physical examination and is confirmed by endoscopy if possible.

2. Surgical consultation if patient on medical service. Medical consultation if on surgical service.

3. Medical treatment proceeds with appropriate blood and fluid replacement, and sedation. Start on acute ulcer diet (milk if tolerated and hourly antacids) for the first 36 to 48 hours, then advance to bland diet and antacids if stable.

4. Patient to remain in hospital for 10 to 14 days.

5. Surgical intervention, as discussed below, if bleeding continues or recurs.

The indications for surgical treatment of patients with bleeding from a peptic ulcer are based on the considerations listed in Table 5-2. As shown in this table, mortality increases sharply in patients with continuing or recurrent hemorrhage especially in older patients. Avery Jones and Gummer (4) have demonstrated that emergency surgical treatment of these patients will reduce sharply their mortality. From 1941 to 1946 surgical treatment was used only as a last resort in 3 of 379 patients under 60 years of age. Mortality of patients with bleeding gastric ulcer was 14.3% and of those with duodenal ulcer was 2.1%. During the years 1955 to 1957 when surgical treatment was regularly employed for patients with continuing or recurrent bleeding, 28 of 300 patients were operated on, and overall mortality fell to 3.2% for gastric and 0% for duodenal ulcer patients. For patients over the age of 60 years, corresponding figures for mortality were 25% and 23% in 1941 to 1946 and 11.5% and 10.5% in 1955 to 1957. Since during this 25-year period the understanding of transfusion and fluid and electrolyte requirements improved greatly, the improved mortality statistics cannot be attributed to the more aggressive surgical approach alone. Nevertheless, there is now general agreement that surgical intervention is appropriate in patients whose bleeding continues or recurs while under medical therapy. The statistics cited above were obtained at a time when subtotal gastrectomy was the standard operative procedure in these patients. More recent experience (24,25) indicates that good control of hemorrhage, as well as acceptable long-term recurrence rates, are attainable with vagotomy and pyloroplasty combined with ligation of the bleeding vessel. This operation is associated with a much lesser surgical mortality than gastrectomy and is, therefore, generally considered the operation of choice in emergency situations. However, there is an increased risk of rebleeding after this operation, and its role in patients with bleeding gastric, as opposed to duodenal ulcer is still unsettled (24). The considerations that enter into the choice of a specific operation will be discussed later in this chapter.

Based on these data, emergency surgical intervention is indicated in any patient bleeding from chronic peptic ulcer whose hemorrhage continues briskly over 6 to 12 hours after admission, or stops and recurs. These considerations apply especially to patients over the age of 50 years, in whom the bleeding has been documented as coming from a chronic peptic ulcer. The operation to be used in these patients must be determined by the surgeon, based on the diagnosis, the patient's condition at the time of operation, and on his experience with the various surgical procedures. Pyloroplasty and truncal vagotomy with oversewing of the bleeding vessel is probably the operation attended by the least mortality.

Patients bleeding from marginal ulcers deserve special comment. Bleeding from marginal ulcers is a relatively rare cause of massive upper gastrointestinal bleeding. Thus Schiller et al (9) reported that these patients accounted for only 0.6% of cases in their series. However, Palmer (14) noted that 29% of such patients came to emergency surgery. Avery Jones (13) reported that 23% of these patients had a second bleeding episode in the hospital. The overall mortality of patients with bleeding marginal ulcer in Avery Jones' series was 6.8% of 112 subjects (13). Schiller et al (9) reported a mortality rate of 31% in 13 patients, a very small series. In these patients consideration must be given to three major causes for recurrent ulceration, each of which requires a different type of definitive surgical treatment. In general, marginal ulcers should be treated by elective surgery, since medical therapy is followed by an unacceptable recurrence rate (26). If clinical conditions permit, before further surgery is undertaken the possibility of Zollinger-Ellison syndrome should be tested for by means of a serum gastrin determination. A high serum gastrin will suggest this diagnosis, but may also be found in patients with retained antral mucosa. This latter diagnosis can, however, be ruled out by review of the original operative note or specimen, if they show the presence of a duodenal cuff on the resected specimen. Incomplete vagotomy can be tested for by the Hollander test. In an emergency situation if the clinical picture suggests Zollinger-Ellison syndrome (marginal ulcer, diarrhea, large amounts of gastric juice with pH < 2), a total gastrectomy may have to be considereed. Hopefully in the near future such patients can be treated with H2 receptor antagonists (27).

The indications for elective surgery in the case of patients with bleeding peptic ulcer are not as clearly defined as those for emergency operations. In general, a single episode of bleeding, especially in a younger patient (less than 50 years of age) with relatively few symptoms of dyspepsia, is not an indication for surgical treatment. However, if such a patient has a rare blood group, or perhaps other problems with transfusions, or some complicating illness that would make another bleeding episode very dangerous, then elective surgical therapy may be considered. By contrast, a patient over the age of 50 years, with a previous history of bleeding from an ulcer, or with severe ulcer dyspepsia or a past history of pyloric obstruction (28) would be seriously considered as a candidate for elective surgery for relief of the ulcer disease. In older patients, those over the age of 75 years, the greater risk of surgery and the greater frequency of intercurrent illness may suggest a more conservative approach. Therefore, we believe the decision about elective surgical treatment must be made individually, based on all the facts for that particular patient and with his or her fully informed agreement.

Stress ulcers and erosive gastritis.   Stress ulceration and erosive gastritis will be treated together in this section, since their etiology, diagnosis, and management are similar. Ulceration in association with other severe disease was first described by Curling in 1842 (29) in patients with severe burns and associated ulceration of the duodenum. Since then a substantial, but confusing, literature has developed on this topic. Stillman and Silen (30) have reviewed the etiologic factors responsible for these syndromes and have suggested that the lesions be considered under four major groups of ulceration based on their postulated pathogenesis. The four groups are as follows.

1. *Curling ulcers.* These are usually large, penetrating ulcers of the duodenum with some fibrosis in the base, occurring several days after a severe burn in about 10% of patients.

2. *Cushing's ulcer.* These ulcers may occur in the esophagus, stomach, or duodenum in patients with cerebral trauma or tumors. First described by Cushing in 1932 (31), they are often large lesions associated with necrosis of the wall of the affected organ.

3. *Drug related ulceration.* These are multiple superficial ulcerations usually seen in the fundus or body of the stomach in association with ingestion of salicylates, phenylbutazone, indomethacin, and alcohol, secondary to drug-induced mucosal injury (32).

4. *Stress ulceration.* These are multiple, acute superficial ulcers or occasionally discrete superficial ulcers without fibrosis, occurring in patients with severe trauma, sepsis, or postoperatively. The common feature in all these cases is severe sepsis (33).

This classification appears useful clinically, since it suggests approaches to therapy and gives some idea of prognosis. The ulceration seen with drug ingestion (Group 3) often produces hemorrhage that, however, fortunately is commonly relatively mild and responds to medical therapy. In contrast, the hemorrhage from stress ulcers (Group 4) is frequently massive and fatal, but may be preventable as discussed below. Curling ulcers, on the other hand, being often single may be more readily managed surgically if bleeding is severe enough to require intervention. Unfortunately, it is not always easy to fit a particular patient into one of these four categories. Thus, Beil et al (34) in reviewing a five-year experience with 35 patients with postoperative gastrointestinal bleeding found that 24 of their patients had solitary ulcers, while 11 had multiple lesions. Harkins (35) had made similar observations based on a review of the literature in 1939. Mears (36) found acute ulcerations at autopsy in 3.8% of burn patients and 7.7% of patients with myocardial infarctions. Nevertheless, the classification described above is useful as a guide to management, especially when the diagnosis can be established by means of panendoscopy or angiography or both (see Chapter 3).

Bleeding from stress ulcers or erosive gastritis accounts for approximately 15% of all cases of upper gastrointestinal hemorrhage (14,15). These lesions, however, become even more prevalent in the group of patients in whom bleeding develops in the hospital, especially in the intensive care unit, as a complication of a major illness. Indeed, in these patients stress ulceration is the major cause of bleeding, and an important cause of death. Recent work (30,37) suggests that many of these lesions may be preventable by intensive antacid therapy, which is aimed at complete neutralization of gastric acid, especially in patients with burns or sepsis. This requires continuous intragastric administration of antacid and monitoring of pH. Although these reports need confirmation, they hold out the promise of preventive therapy for a very dangerous problem. If upper gastrointestinal bleeding nevertheless develops in a patient in hospital, especially if the hospital course has been complicated by severe sepsis or shock, a diagnosis of stress ulceration must be considered. In patients presenting to the hospital with hemorrhage and a history of drug ingestion or alcohol abuse, a diagnosis of erosive gastritis is very likely (see Chapter 2). The investigation of these patients should then proceed as outlined in Schemes 2-1 and 2-2 (Chapter 2). If technically feasible, panendoscopy should be carried out, as this will permit a precise diagnosis to be made. In particular, it will differentiate between a diffuse erosive gastritis and a localized ulcer, and thus allow the medical-surgical team to plan appropriate therapy. If endoscopy is not possible because of continued bleeding or other reasons, selective abdominal arteriography may localize the site of bleeding and, if indicated, provide a means of controlling bleeding by intraarterial infusion of pitressin (Chapters 3,5).

Despite these measures, however, patients with erosive gastritis and stress ulceration do frequently suffer massive bleeding and thus present serious problems in management. When this happens, the indications for surgical intervention are similar to those in patients with peptic ulcers, that is, continuing or recurrent overt hemorrhage despite intensive medical therapy. There is no agreement at present on the type of operation best suited to the management of these patients. Menguy, Gadatz, and Zatchuk (38), and Luke and Dragstedt (39) have reported very high recurrence rates of hemorrhage following pyloroplasty and vagotomy or partial gastrectomy with gastrojejunostomy, with or without vagotomy, and, therefore, suggest high subtotal gastric resection (80%-90%) as the operation of choice. Desmond and Reynolds (40) reported their experience with 331 patients with erosive gastritis over 30 years. Of these patients, 47 came to emergency surgery mainly in the last 5 years of the study. These authors found that best results were obtained with partial gastrectomy and gastroduodenostomy. Of the 28 patients who underwent this operation, only one had a recurrence of bleeding needing further surgery, and there were five deaths. The other procedures had recurrence rates of about 50%, in line with the findings of others (38,39). Desmond and Reynolds emphasized the value of immediate endoscopy for defining the precise anatomic diagnosis, followed by early surgical treatment. More recently, Athanasoulis and co-workers (41) have had good results in controlling bleeding in such patients with intraarterial infusion of pitressin. Only 4 of 37 patients so treated required surgical therapy. Our own experience with a smaller number of patients has also been encouraging.

The situation is somewhat different in those patients in whom endoscopy shows a solitary ulcer in the stomach or duodenum without diffuse erosive gastritis. In these patients, pyloroplasty and vagotomy with ligation of the bleeding vessel offers a good chance of controlling the bleeding, but high recurrence rates for bleeding have been reported (38). However, even in these patients selective intraarterial infusion of pitressin may be the preferred method of treatment if the general condition of the patient or the severity of the underlying problem make surgical management hazardous.

We believe, therefore, that patients presenting with hematemesis or melena following ingestion of ulcerogenic drugs or alcohol, or following severe trauma

or shock, should have upper gastrointestinal panendoscopy on an emergency
basis if this can be safely done. If this is not possible, selective abdominal arteriography should be carried out. If bleeding continues despite intensive medical therapy, and the bleeding is due to a diffuse erosive gastritis, selective intraarterial infusion of pitressin should be tried. If this fails, surgical treatment is
indicated. However, the choice of operation at present is not clearly defined. If
endoscopy shows a localized ulcer, pyloroplasty with vagotomy and ligation of
the bleeding vessel is probably the treatment of choice, while multiple ulcerations require high subtotal or total gastrectomy.

Esophageal varices (Scheme 5-1).   The management of patients presenting
with hematemesis or melena complicating hepatic cirrhosis due to whatever
cause presents many major problems. Perhaps the most difficult question to
resolve in these patients is whether the bleeding is actually coming from
esophageal varices (14). For example, among 1000 patients with cirrhosis described by Brick and Palmer, 266 bled from varices, while in 319 hemorrhage
was due to another lesion, of which the most common was duodenal ulcer (109
patients) (42). It is evident from that type of data that the selection of the
appropriate surgical procedure must be based on precise diagnosis, which can
best be obtained by endoscopy (14). Failure to establish the actual source of
bleeding can lead to performance of an emergency shunt only to have the
patient have a further, fatal hemorrhage from a peptic ulcer (43). The other
major problem in the selection of patients for shunt surgery concerns the evaluation of hepatic functional status (44,45). There is significant disagreement and
uncertainty on this important point among different investigators. Other problems include the disorders of clotting function so often seen in patients with
cirrhosis, the multiple metabolic derangements, and the nutritional deficiencies
that complicate their condition.

The approach to the management of the patient with cirrhosis and upper
gastrointestinal bleeding is outlined in Scheme 5-1. A diagnosis of probable
cirrhosis of the liver can usually be established on the basis of a history of excess
alcohol ingestion, or preceding hepatic or biliary disease and the presence of
stigmata of liver disease (enlarged liver, spider angiomata, liver palms, etc). A
preliminary evaluation of the patient in terms of overall hepatic function can
also be made on clinical grounds. The presence of obvious ascites, or jaundice, or
evidence of a bleeding tendency, or of hepatic encephalopathy, suggest advanced liver failure due to either end stage cirrhosis or active liver disease, such
as acute alcoholic hepatitis or chronic active hepatitis. Such findings indicate a
very poor risk patient, who will be unlikely to be able to withstand a major
surgical procedure. However, a final judgment on the patient's eligibility for
possible surgical treatment should not be made until the necessary laboratory
data are available (see below). At this stage, several sources of hemorrhage must
be considered. The most important of these are esophageal varices, erosive
gastritis, peptic ulcer, and deficiency of coagulation factors secondary to liver
disease (see Chapter 2). In addition to the usual measures aimed at replacement
of circulating volume and of red cells, these patients should be given fresh
frozen plasma and vitamin K parenterally after baseline studies have been obtained (Chapter 2). Treatment for actual or impending hepatic encephalopathy

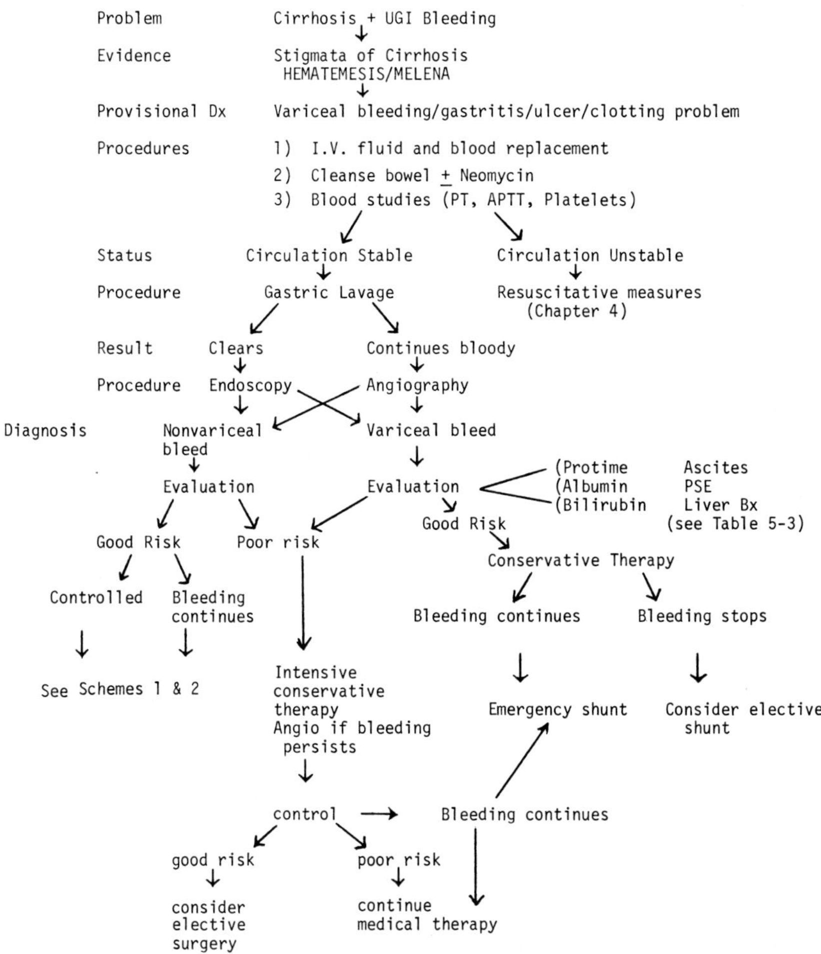

SCHEME 5-1

must be started with cleansing enemas, oral or rectal neomycin, or lactulose, and oral or nasogastric magnesium sulfate.

As in other forms of overt gastrointestinal bleeding the sequence of further diagnostic tests must depend on the circulatory status of the patient (Scheme 5-1). If this is unstable, resuscitative measures as described in Chapter 4 must take precedence. Once these are successful, or if the patient's condition permits, gastric lavage should be performed. In patients in whom lavage fails to clear blood from the stomach, and who, therefore, are continuing to bleed, selective abdominal arteriography should be performed if possible. If, however, gastric contents can be cleared of blood, panendoscopy should be performed to ascertain the source of bleeding. If this shows varices that are still bleeding or that are covered by blood clot, a diagnosis of variceal hemorrhage is made. In the absence of such findings a careful search must be made for gastritis or peptic ulcer. If one of these is found to be the cause of bleeding, the patient should be managed as described in the preceding sections of this chapter, with decisions for or against surgical intervention based on the criteria discussed in those sections. These decisions, however, may require modification based on the results of the evaluation of the patient's hepatic status. These considerations are discussed in more detail below in relation to patients shown to be bleeding from varices.

Once a diagnosis of bleeding from esophageal or gastric varices has been established by endoscopy or angiography, the evaluation of the functional status of the liver must be completed. These studies must be carried out as quickly as possible, and certainly withhin the first 12 to 24 hours after admission (43,45). Various authors differ as to the studies needed to classify patients into good risk, moderate, or bad risk groups (45). In addition to the clinical findings listed earlier and in Table 5-3, three laboratory studies are generally thought to be valuable. They are the serum bilirubin, serum albumin, and the prothrombin time. If the physical signs of liver disease are minimal and the laboratory data near normal, the patient can be considered a good risk for surgery, if this is deemed necessary. Indeed, in Mickelsen's experience all 18 good risk patients survived emergency portacaval shunt surgery (46). On the other hand, patients with gross signs of hepatic failure clinically and by laboratory evaluation are likely to have very high mortality rates with surgical treatment and may need to be managed conservatively, even though the results of such therapy are most discouraging.

The available means for the conservative treatment of the poor risk patient with bleeding varices are limited. Baum and co-workers (47) have reported encouraging results with pitressin infusion through the superior mesenteric artery in these patients. They noted, however, that care must be taken with these patients to guard against water intoxication and hyponatremia due to the antidiuretic effect of the pitressin that enters the systemic circulation. Intraarterial pitressin is thus a hopeful innovation in the management of these extremely ill patients, but a final evaluation of its role in therapy must await further controlled trials. Intravenous pitressin is still recommended by some authors (48). However, it is generally accepted that pitressin used in this way gives only temporary control of bleeding and is, therefore, of very limited value (48). Most recently,

Table 5-3
Evaluation of Hepatic Status

	Good Risk	*Moderate Risk*	*Bad Risk*
Clinical Findings			
Ascites	Minimal	Moderate	Tense
Encephalopathy	±	+ → + +	> + +
Nutritional state	Good	Fair	Poor
Laboratory Data			
Bilirubin mg/100 ml	< 3.0	3.0–6.0	> 6.0
Albumin g/100 ml	> 3.4	2.5–3.4	< 2.5
Prothrombin time seconds (control = 12)	< 15	15–17	> 18

attempts have been made to control variceal bleeding by means of percutaneous injection of sclerosing solution into the varices via portal venous cannulae. Esophageal and gastric tamponade with balloons is still employed, usually using a Sengstaken-Blakemore tube. Conn, in 1959, showed that use of this type of tube is attended by a very high incidence of complications such as aspiration pneumonia and esophageal erosions (49). Use of tamponade should, therefore, be restricted to situations where temporary control of bleeding is a first step to getting a patient ready for more definitive therapy, or to patients for whom no other alternative therapy is available. These conservative measures, however, can only be used for relatively short periods of time. Pitressin infusion, as discussed in Chapter 5, can only be continued for 24 to 48 hours. Similarly, balloon tamponade for periods in excess of 24 to 36 hours is associated with a rapidly rising complication rate (49). While these measures to control variceal bleeding are being carried out alone or in combination, a full evaluation of the coagulation factors should be performed and appropriate replacement therapy should be instituted in consultation with the Hematology service. Such replacement therapy will usually consist of fresh frozen plasma and vitamin K. In special circumstances, where a fibrinolytic syndrome or intravascular coagulation are present, treatment with epsilon amino caproic acid or heparin may be considered (50).

If the patient is judged to be in the good or moderate risk group, the question of surgical treatment must be carefully considered. The first decision to be made is whether surgical therapy is indicated and if so, whether emergency surgery is to be undertaken, or whether elective surgery is to be preferred. The second decision concerns the type of surgical procedure to be performed. There is no general agreement on the answers to any of these questions. Indeed, even with the data from randomized controlled studies of elective shunt surgery available (44,51,52), the value of therapeutic shunts is not fully established. The studies reported by Mickelsen (44) and Jackson (51) suggest better survival of patients randomized to elective portacaval shunt than of patients randomized to medical therapy. However, in the latter study the best survival rate was attained by the small group of patients randomized to surgical treatment but who refused portacaval shunt (51). Seven of these 11 patients (63.6%) survived an average of 5½ years, in contrast to 37 of 67 (55%) of patients operated on (51). Survival in the medically treated group was 37% (19 of 51). Resnick (52), reporting on the Boston study, concluded that there was no statistical advantage in survival in the shunted patients compared with the medically treated group (56% v. 48%). There is somewhat better agreement on the value of emergency shunt surgery (43,46). Thus, immediate survival in patients bleeding massively from varices with failure to control bleeding within 12 to 24 hours was only 17% with medical therapy, compared with 53% in the patients treated by emergency shunt surgery, while at 4 years the corresponding figures were 3% and 40% respectively (43). Some authorities recommend transesophageal ligation of varices as the emergency operation of choice (48); however, this is a minority view.

Patient selection for surgical treatment is still a problem. Mikkelsen (44) believes a liver biopsy must be obtained preoperatively and surgery postponed if this shows acute alcoholic hepatitis. Other contraindications to elective shunt surgery are advanced age (>60 years), episodes of hepatic encephalopathy, and poor liver function (Table 5-3) (45). However, these are general guidelines and decisions must be made on an individual basis. Our own experience supports the value of emergency portacaval shunts in patients with uncontrolled or recurrent variceal bleeding, who are in the good or moderate risk groups. The question of elective shunts remains unresolved. We agree with Mikkelsen (44) that a liver biopsy should be obtained prior to surgery. If this shows acute alcoholic liver disease, and the patient is stable, it is worth waiting for several weeks, since with resolution of the acute process the varices may disappear (42). Furthermore, the prognosis of patients with post-hepatitic or cryptogenic cirrhosis as a group is poor with shunt surgery (45). Therefore, a final decision should at least in part be based on a firm histologic diagnosis.

Careful studies (53,54) have established that there is no place for prophylactic shunts in the management of patients with alcoholic cirrhosis. Therefore, this procedure should never be performed. We believe emergency portacaval shunt is a valuable lifesaving procedure in patients with uncontrolled variceal bleeding, whose liver function is adequate (good, or moderate risk groups). Since the three randomized studies of therapeutic shunts have failed to show a statistically significant increase in survival with shunt surgery, the value of this operation must be judged by the quality of life of the survivors. In this respect, both the Veterans study (51) and the Boston study (52) suggest that the surgically treated patients do better. Thus, the rehospitalization rate for the medically treated group in the Boston study was 130%, while that of the surgically treated patients was only 63%. Therefore, in a patient with acceptable hepatic function, under the age of 60, we believe elective shunt surgery has a place.

Mallory Weiss syndrome (Schemes 2-1 and 2-2).   After it was first described by Mallory and Weiss in 1929, this syndrome was considered to be a rare and frequently fatal disorder. However, with the advent of endoscopy it was recognized to be quite a common cause of hematemesis. Palmer (14) found esophageal mucosal tears in 5.7% of 1400 patients presenting with upper gastrointestinal bleeding. Furthermore, it became apparent that the majority of patients with this condition had relatively mild episodes of hemorrhage, which most often proved self-limiting. Alcoholic gastritis was thought to be the most frequent precipitating factor. Saylor and Tedesco (55) found this syndrome to be the cause of hematemesis in over 10% of their series of patients, and observed that alcohol abuse was the initiating factor in less than half of their patients. Other associated factors included salicylates and antral gastritis. The great majority of their patients recovered with conservative management. Only in rare instances did bleeding continue, or recur, and require more aggressive therapy.

The diagnosis is usually suggested by the history of repeated dry heaves followed ultimately by hematemesis. It is readily confirmed by endoscopic examination, which reveals a linear mucosal tear in the region of the esophagogastric junction. In the typical case, treatment with a soft or liquid diet, antacids, and transfusion if necessary, is adequate. Rarely hemorrhage may be more severe and continuous. In such cases, intraarterial infusion of pitressin via the left gastric or superior mesenteric artery, depending on which vessel is the source of bleeding, will usually control the situation (41). In rare instances surgical repair of the esophageal tear is necessary. This will clearly be necessary in the unusual case where a total esophageal tear with perforation into the mediastinum has occurred (Boerhave's syndrome). This situation can readily be suspected on clinical grounds because of the presence of severe retrosternal pain and subcutaneous emphysema in the root of the neck or the epigastrium. The diagnosis can then be confirmed by radiography of the chest. If this diagnosis is suspected, endoscopy should not be performed. In case of doubt, an esophagogram using an iodide containing dye can be used for confirmation. Treatment is immediate surgical drainage of the mediastinum and repair of the esophageal tear if this is judged safe. In cases seen some hours after the event mediastinal drainage alone should be done, and a feeding gastrostomy tube should be inserted.

Other causes of upper gastrointestinal bleeding.   The diagnosis of peptic ulcer, gastritis, esophageal varices, and Mallory-Weiss syndrome as causes of upper gastrointestinal bleeding is fairly straightforward. It is the decision for or against surgical treatment of these conditions that creates problems for the physician caring for the patient. The situation is reversed with the other causes of hematemesis or melena listed in Table 2-2. These conditions, and carcinoma of the stomach, clearly fall into two categories, namely those in which surgical removal of the lesion is the only effective therapy, and those for which there is no surgical therapy, or surgery is absolutely contraindicated. The problem in many of these disorders rests in establishing the diagnosis. Stress ulcers and erosive gastritis have already been discussed (Chapter 5, pp. 65–68).

Aortic aneurysms with aorto-enteric fistula and *mesenteric vascular occlusions* present absolute indications for immediate surgical intervention once the diagnosis is established. The diagnosis must be suspected on clinical grounds as discussed in Chapter 2. The diagnosis may be confirmed by arteriography if the patient's condition permits, but it may be dangerous in cases with an aneurysm. Nowadays most instances of aorto-enteric (usually duodenal) fistulae occur at the site of aortic grafts. Gastrointestinal bleeding in patients with such a graft should always raise the suspicion of an aorto-enteric fistula. Therefore, the decision for immediate laparotomy in most cases must be based on clinical judgment. For the patient with a leaking aneurysm, removal of the diseased segment of the aorta, with placement of a graft is the appropriate treatment. In patients with mesenteric vascular occlusion, removal of the dead bowel is mandatory. If the occlusion is due to an embolus, embolectomy may be possible if the patient is seen early enough. In many patients a second look operation should be performed after 24 hours to ascertain viability of the remaining bowel.

The diagnosis of *arteriovenous malformations* depends essentially on selective abdominal arteriography at the time of active bleeding. Not uncommonly a definitive diagnosis is not made until after several episodes of hemorrhage. Once the lesion is demonstrated, surgical removal should be undertaken. *Tumors of the stomach* are usually readily diagnosed by endoscopy or barium contrast studies. *Carcinoma of the stomach* is a rare cause of major bleeding (Table 2-1). Whenever possible, it should be resected. *Leiomyoma* and *leiomyosarcomas* of the stomach are rare tumors which, however, usually present with a major hemorrhage. Once the diagnosis is made by endoscopy or barium studies, surgical removal of the lesion is indicated. *Adenomatous polyps* of the stomach are almost uniformly benign and do not usually cause overt hemorrhage. They may cause chronic occult blood loss and, if so, may require surgical removal. *Benign and malignant tumors* of the duodenum and small bowel are rare tumors and will be discussed further in Chapter 6. The diagnosis usually is made by careful barium contrast studies of the small bowel or by arteriography. Surgical removal of the lesion is the only effective therapy. *Hemobilia* usually results from a tumor of the biliary tree, aneurysm of the hepatic artery, or trauma to the liver or biliary tree. The diagnosis is strongly suggested by the history of biliary colic followed by bleeding, relief of pain, and then appearance of jaundice, which may be mild or transient, and melena. Hematemesis is less common. Surgical exploration is indicated.

The importance of the *heredofamilial disorders* that involve the gastrointestinal tract and result in hemorrhage lies in the fact that, although rare, they cause recurring episodes of bleeding. The diagnosis is usually readily established by careful review of the family history and meticulous physical examination, which will reveal the pathognomonic findings listed in Table 2-2. The diagnosis can be confirmed by skin biopsy in patients with pseudoxanthoma elasticum or Ehlers-Danlos syndrome, and by endoscopic observation of telengiectasia of the gastric mucosa in patients with that disease. The common major causes of upper gastrointestinal hemorrhage must be ruled out by appropriate studies, and the patient must be treated with blood replacement and iron supplements as necessary. The *hematologic disorders* are diagnosed by appropriate studies of coagulation factors and should be referred to a hematologist for long-term management. The management of patients with *disseminated intravascular coagulation* or *fibrinolytic syndrome* has already been discussed (Chapter 5, pp.71). Withdrawal of the offending drug is the treatment in patients bleeding due to toxic effects of medications. Parenteral administration of vitamin K is indicated in patients bleeding from an *overdose of anticoagulants*. If the bleeding is massive, immediate replacement therapy with fresh frozen plasma or clotting factor concentrates may be necessary.

Lower intestinal bleeding (Scheme 2-3)

Life threatening hemorrhage from the small-bowel distal to the ligament of Treitz and the large bowel is uncommon. When this occurs, as discussed in Chapters 2 and 3, selective arteriography is the best means of localizing the bleeding site, unless that procedure is contraindicated by the extent of vascular disease or iodide sensitivity. Once a bleeding site is identified, the patient should be prepared for surgical exploration and removal of the lesion.

More commonly, however, intestinal bleeding is less severe and investigation of the patient can proceed as discussed previously (Chapter 2). If the patient is seen at a time when active bleeding is still going on, especially if the patient has a previous history of hemorrhage without a firm diagnosis as to site, and rectal examination, with or without sigmoidoscopy have not established a diagnosis, selective arteriography is probably indicated (47,56). This procedure can localize the site of bleeding in many instances and thus can help to define which of perhaps multiple abnormalities, such as hiatus hernia and diverticular disease, is the source of the problem. More often, however, with lower intestinal bleeding this will have stopped by the time the patient is seen and, therefore, angiography is less urgent and less likely to be helpful. In this situation it is best to proceed with a barium enema, followed by an upper gastrointestinal series and small-bowel examination. If these are negative and history suggests colonic bleeding, colonoscopy may be helpful. In patients under the age of 25 and without obvious clinical findings, the possibility of a *Meckel's diverticulum* should be considered. Rutherford and Akers in a review of 148 children with Meckel's diverticulum noted that typically hemorrhage in their patients was recurrent and painless (57). Most often, bright red blood was passed per rectum. A pertechnitate scan can be used to confirm this diagnosis in some cases. If these studies fail to make a diagnosis, and bleeding has stopped, the patient is classified as an undiagnosed bleeder and further management should proceed as described in Chapter 6. If bleeding is continuing or has recurred in face of negative findings, angiography should be undertaken; and if a bleeding site is identified, this should be treated surgically.

In most patients with lower intestinal bleeding, one of the diagnoses listed in Table 2-3 will be identified by the usual investigations. The problem then is to determine whether the lesion found is the cause of bleeding. The finding of a *carcinoma of the colon* is an absolute indication for resection of the lesion even if only a palliative resection is possible. It is important to bear in mind that, like gastric carcinomas, cancers of the colon rarely bleed massively. Therefore, in the unusual case of a patient with a malignant tumor in the colon and massive bleeding a careful search for an alternative source of the hemorrhage must be carried out. If another lesion is found, appropriate treatment, which may also be surgical, has to be planned to take into account both conditions.

Diverticular disease of the colon presents a particularly difficult problem in management of intestinal bleeding. As is discussed in Chapter 2, major hemorrhage from diverticula occurs in only about 5% of patients with this disease (58,59,60). Since, however, diverticula are found in 30% of subjects over the age of 60 years (61), the lesion will be frequently encountered in patients with intestinal bleeding. Proof that bleeding is originating from the diverticulum may be difficult to obtain. If it is sufficiently active bleeding (1-2 cc/min), arteriography may show the site (Chapter 3). It is currently believed that this is more likely to come from the right side of the colon than the left (47,56). If the bleeding has stopped or slowed, colonoscopy may help to define the site of bleeding. However, very often a definitive identification of the bleeding site is not possible in these patients. Unless the hemorrhage has been massive, a decision to resect the affected portion of the colon must rest on the extent to which the disease is interfering with the patient's life, on the anatomic extent of the disease, and the presence or absence of other complications, such as pericolic abscess. If surgical treatment is indicated on these grounds, the episode of bleeding would reinforce this decision. If, however, there are no other indications for surgery than the bleeding episode, surgery may be postponed until more definitive proof that the diverticular disease is responsible for the bleeding is obtained. In the case of a patient with massive bleeding from the colon and diffuse diverticular disease, most surgeons favor colectomy.

Inflammatory bowel disease, that is, ulcerative colitis and Crohn's disease frequently present as rectal bleeding. In one series (62), patients with these two diseases accounted for 25% of all cases of rectal hemorrhage. Massive or life threatening hemorrhage is fortunately a rare complication of these diseases (63,64). The diagnosis of inflammatory bowel disease can usually be readily established on clinical grounds and sigmoidoscopic examination and can be confirmed by barium contrast studies once the patient's condition is stable. In rare instances, especially with ulcerative colitis, massive bleeding may require emergency colectomy. In these cases, there is usually little doubt about the diagnosis after clinical and sigmoidoscopic examination. A plain radiograph of the abdomen will often help confirm the diagnosis by showing either toxic dilatation of the colon, or a grossly irregular colonic outline indicating pseudopolyposis. Unless such an emergency situation exists, the patient should be treated medically. Treatment will consist of a low residue or liquid diet, adrenocorticosteroids or salazo-sulfapyridine, blood transfusions, and rest. Indications for elective surgical treatment of these conditions are based on the severity, duration, and extent of the disease, and on the presence or absence of extra-enteric complications (63,64).

Polyps of the colon, small-bowel tumors, hemorrhoids, and *anal fissures* very rarely cause major hemorrhage. Polyps and small-bowel tumors, if found in the course of evaluating a patient with intestinal bleeding, should be removed either endoscopically or surgically depending on size and location. If no other lesion is detected, it is likely that the bleeding was due to the neoplasm. However, the patient should be carefully followed, both for evidence of recurrence of the lesion or of bleeding. Hemorrhoids and anal fissures can usually be treated by control of constipation or diarrhea, and local application of medication. Surgical removal may be necessary for symptoms other than bleeding, although rarely this may lead to operation.

Vascular malformations of the large and small bowel have become more readily recognized with the advent of arteriography. Angiodysplasia of the right colon has been shown to occur, particularly in older subjects with arteriosclerotic heart disease (47,56). In most cases, bleeding is chronic rather than massive and, therefore, will rarely require emergency surgical intervention. Once the diagnosis is established, elective removal of the lesion is indicated. Other *vascular malformations* such as hemangiomata, arteriovenous fistulae, and telangiectasis are rare lesions. Thus McHardy and colleagues (65) found no examples of these conditions among 88 personal cases of bleeding from the small bowel. This is probably an underestimate, since this series was studied before arteriography was available. With availability of this means of investigation, vascular lesions are more frequently recognized. When such a lesion is demonstrated surgical, excision is the treatment of choice. Infarction of the region of the splenic flexure of the colon due to *occlusion of the inferior mesenteric artery* is another rare condition. Occlusion of this artery occurs fairly frequently without colonic infarction. When infarction does occur, it may present as an acute abdominal catastrophe, usually in elderly patients. The rectum is preserved. The diagnosis is usually made at laparotomy. Resection of the infarcted bowel is the treatment. In some cases, however, the infarction may develop insidiously (called ischemic colitis) and present with abdominal pain and signs of low-grade obstruction or chronic bleeding. The diagnosis can be made by barium enema with the characteristic distribution of loss of mucosal pattern and thumbprinting and narrowing involving the distal transverse colon, splenic flexure, and proximal descending colon. In this case, conservative management is indicated.

Occult gastrointestinal bleeding (Scheme 2-4)

Occult bleeding from the digestive tract is a common cause of chronic iron deficiency anemia. The approach to the investigation of patients with this problem has been reviewed in Chapter 2. The treatment of the problem once the causative lesion has been identified is not usually a major problem. The difficult part of management in this situation is ascertaining the cause of chronic blood loss. Many of the abnormalities of the digestive tract revealed by barium contrast studies are common disorders, often occurring in otherwise asymptomatic individuals. Therefore, it is necessary that the physician satisfy himself that the lesion found by full clinical and radiologic evaluation of the patient is the cause of bleeding.

Hiatus hernia is commonly accepted as a cause of gastrointestinal blood loss. If the patient has definite symptoms of reflux, heartburn, or dysphagia and occult blood in the stool, it is reasonable to consider the hiatal hernia as the probable cause. However, other lesions must be ruled out by careful clinical evaluation and by appropriate radiologic studies. It should be remembered that hiatus hernia by itself is not a cause of bleeding. Only when it is complicated by esophagitis or ulceration is that the case. Therefore, an upper gastrointestinal endoscopy should be performed to document the presence of esophagitis and to evaluate the status of the stomach and duodenum. In cases of doubt, an esophageal biopsy should be obtained. Once the diagnosis is established, a trial of medical therapy is in order unless the esophagitis is of great severity, or unless an actual stricture is present. An associated duodenal ulcer also makes the prognosis with medical therapy less promising. Medical therapy will include weight reduction, if the patient is overweight, antacids, frequent small meals, and elevation of the head of the bed. If medical therapy fails to control the problem, or one of the complications is present, surgical repair of the hernia will be indicated. Current surgical practice is to repair the hernia and to perform a fundoplication. If a peptic ulcer is also present, the surgical approach should include a procedure for controlling the ulcer disease. There is still no general agreement on the best procedure for this purpose. Parietal cell or selective vagotomy, truncal vagotomy and pyloroplasty and Billroth I gastrectomy with vagotomy all have their advocates.

Diverticular disease as indicated earlier is a common disorder in older patients and can be the cause of occult bleeding. However, it is often an incidental finding. Therefore, as with hiatus hernia, a careful clinical and radiologic search for other sources of bleeding is mandatory before diverticular disease can be accepted as the source. Indeed, in a patient with persistent occult bleeding and colonic diverticula the possibility of a carcinoma of the colon must be borne in mind. It may be very difficult for the radiologist to rule out this possibility with confidence. In such cases, therefore, colonoscopy should be considered to rule out this condition. If no cancer is present, and other causes of bleeding are ruled out, treatment should generally be conservative with stool softeners, antispasmodics, and a normal diet. Surgical removal of the diseased bowel is indicated only if the patient's symptoms are troublesome and not responsive to medical measures.

Probably the most common cause of occult bleeding is the ingestion of *salicylates*. The approach to this problem was fully reviewed in Chapter 2. The treatment consists of withdrawal of the drug, if possible, once its etiologic relationship to bleeding has been documented (Chapter 2). *Peptic ulcer* and *esophageal varices* may cause occult bleeding. In the case of peptic ulcer disease this should respond to medical therapy. Surgical treatment of the ulcer will be indicated only if the ulcer proves resistant to these measures. In the case of the patient with varices and occult bleeding, treatment should be aimed at avoidance of precipitating factors, such as alcohol abuse, or salicylates. Shunt surgery should be reserved for patients with major hemorrhage as discussed under the second section of this chapter (Specific Disease States: Upper Gastrointestinal Bleeding).

Benign or malignant tumors of the gastrointestinal tract will often present with occult bleeding. Once they are identified by radiologic and endoscopic means, they should be removed surgically if at all possible. *Vascular malformations*, including telangiectasia, arteriovenous fistulae, and angiodysplasia (Table 2-2) are rare causes of bleeding. However, occult bleeding is a common manifestation of these conditions. Localized malformations should be treated by surgical resection. Diffuse lesions, such as telangiectasia, are not amenable to excision. Patients with this type of lesion will require therapy with iron supplements and transfusions as necessary, and reassurance.

Hereditary disorders such as Peutz-Jeghers syndrome, pseudoxanthoma elasticum, and Ehlers-Danlos syndrome may also present with occult bleeding. Treatment again consists of iron and blood replacement and reassurance. As indicated in Chapter 2, patients with occult bleeding should be evaluated from the point of view of disorders of hemostasis. If one of these disorders is found, appropriate therapy must be instituted.

INTRAARTERIAL INFUSION THERAPY

Arteriography as it relates to the identification of the site of bleeding is discussed in Chapter 3. In this section, we review the current status of intraarterial infusion of pharmacologic agents in the management of patients with gastrointestinal hemorrhage. This form of therapy is thought to be most helpful in three groups of patients. First, those in whom surgical management is contraindicated because of some intercurrent medical problems, such as a very recent myocardial infarction; second, those in whom operative intervention may be rendered unnecessary, as for example in patients with bleeding from diverticular disease of the colon, and third, those in whom an emergency operation would carry a grave prognosis, which would be much improved if an operation could be performed electively. Intraarterial infusion of therapeutic agents, therefore, may be a valuable addition to our therapeutic armamentarium in selected patients, in whom the site of hemorrhage has been defined by endoscopic or angiographic means. The optimal selection of patients for this form of therapy has not yet been fully defined. In a review of experience from the Boston City Hospital, Byrne et al (66) reported that among 172 patients without cirrhosis with massive hemorrhage from sources other than esophageal varices, the mortality was 25%, whereas 37.5% of 56 patients with cirrhosis and nonvariceal bleeding died. In a similar group of patients with cirrhosis of the liver and nonvariceal bleeding, Wirthlin et al (67) reported a mortality of 57% following emergency surgical treatment, compared with a 9% fatality rate in patients operated on electively. Thus the risks of surgical treatment are, at least in part determined by factors other than the actual site of bleeding, and they may be influenced by the timing of the operation. Even temporary control of bleeding by means of intraarterial infusion therapy, by allowing time for the restoration of the circulatory and biochemical status of the patient, may greatly improve the chances of successful management. Table 5-4 presents data collected from the literature to illustrate the success rates for control of hemorrhage by selective intraarterial pitressin infusion, depending on the nature of the bleeding site. In several instances the control of hemorrhage was only temporary, and bleeding recurred following cessation of pitressin infusion. Several reports have demonstrated the complete or partial success of this method of treatment (68-75). Despite this, the precise place of intraarterial vasopressin in the management of patients with massive upper gastrointestinal bleeding is not yet clarified. Conn et al (76) have reported their experience with a controlled, randomized study of this form of therapy in 53 patients with 60 major bleeding episodes due to a variety of lesions. Although intraarterial vasopressin therapy proved significantly more effective in controlling hemorrhage from both varices and other lesions than conventional therapy, and reduced the requirement for blood transfusion, overall survival in this group of patients was not improved by vasopressin infusion. It may be, therefore, that there is a need for better definition of those groups of patients who are most likely to benefit from this form of treatment. In our own experience it has proved most valuable in controlling hemorrhage from stress ulceration and erosive gastritis, but it has been of only limited usefulness in patients bleeding from chronic peptic ulcers and esophageal varices.

The value of intraarterial pitressin infusion in the treatment of patients with lower gastrointestinal bleeding has been more clearly established. Angiographic techniques have now demonstrated that major bleeding from colonic

Table 5-4

Lesion	*No. of Patients*	*Stopped Bleeding with Pitressin*	*Percentage of Pitressin "Effective"*
Duodenal ulcer	43	19	44
Varices	107	59	55
Mallory-Weiss	7	7	100
Gastritis	109	90	83
Gastric ulcer	5	5	100
Colonic diverticula	26	25	96
Inflammatory bowel	3	3	100
AV Malformation	2	2	100
Miscellaneous	19	11	58

(Compiled from References 68, 69, 72, 73, 75, 76, 78, 80, 86).

diverticula occurs preponderantly from the right side of the colon (77,78,79). This observation has allowed for more rapid and more direct surgical intervention in such patients. Furthermore, recent reports strongly support the apparent efficacy of intraarterial infusion of pitressin for the control of bleeding from this lesion (78,79). Further studies may well prove this approach to be the treatment of choice for diverticular hemorrhage.

Although pitressin is the drug most frequently used in clinical practice, earlier experience included the usage of epinephrine, angiotensin (80), growth hormone (81), and propranolol and epinephrine combined. Autologous clot and gelfoam have also been used, although in a limited number of patients. Pitressin was originally given by slow injection into a peripheral vein, but this was found to have a high incidence of serious adverse effects such as hypertension, bradycardia and arrhythmias. Since the introduction of intraarterial pitressin infusion, these complications have occurred with lower frequency, and the expected problems of oliguria, water retention, and hyponatremia have been said not to cause major difficulties if careful attention is paid to water and electrolyte balance during the infusion (82). This question is of particular importance in cirrhotic patients, in whom the infused pitressin may escape removal by the liver and, therefore, may lead to water intoxication. The half-life of pitressin in dog experiments was 5 to 6 minutes and was estimated at 7 to 8 minutes in man (83). Nevertheless, serum sodium levels should be regularly monitored in all patients with pitressin infusion to guard against this complication.

The possibility of inducing bowel ischemia with prolonged selective arterial catheterization was seriously considered at one time (84). But further experience has shown that the catheter itself could be left in place for several days, provided that it was not wedged into the artery, and that backflow of injected contrast material can be demonstrated (85). The fear that pitressin itself might disrupt the gastric mucosal barrier during left gastric or celiac artery infusions, and thus actually worsen the hemorrhage, has been shown to be groundless. Another source of concern has been the potential induction of hepatic ischemia, by infusion of pitressin into the hepatic arterial supply. This could happen with either celiac artery infusions or, in rare instances, where the hepatic artery comes off the superior mesenteric artery, in patients being so treated for bleeding esophageal varices. To avoid this problem, it is advisable to advance the catheter beyond the take off of the hepatic artery in patients in whom infusion of the left gastric or gastroduodenal artery is desired. In superior mesenteric artery infusions a dye injection to outline the hepatic arterial blood supply should be carried out (86). In fact, incidental infusion of both normal and cirrhotic livers, without apparent adverse effects up to 8 hours, has been reported (56). However, Marubbio et al (86) have reported one instance where hepatic ischemia was produced.

Once the decision has been made to use intraarterial pitressin infusion therapy in a patient with upper gastrointestinal bleeding, the first requirement for success is selective catheterization of the artery supplying the bleeding lesion. In the case of a gastric ulcer or erosions, this will usually be the left gastric artery; for duodenal ulcers it will usually be the pancreaticoduodenal artery, and, in patients with bleeding esophageal varices, the superior mesenteric artery. Initially, a bolus of 0.5 to 1.0 units of pitressin should be injected, and the response of the vessel in question should be checked by further dye injection. If the artery

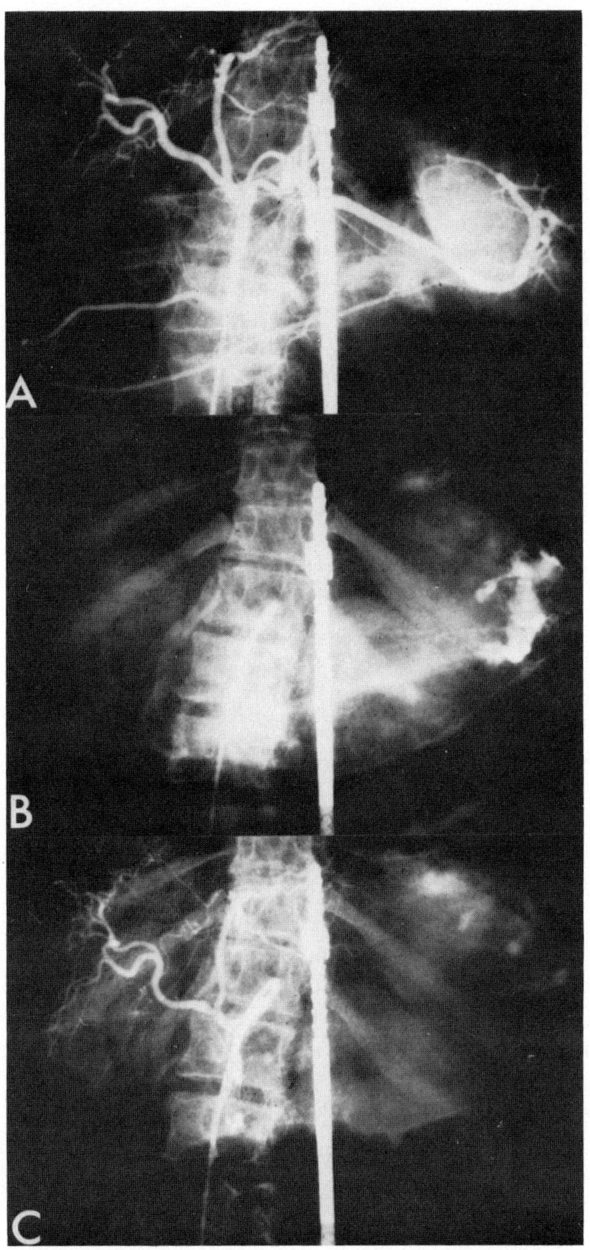

FIGURE 5-1

Left gastric arteriogram in a patient with severe sepsis secondary to spinal surgery. Hematemesis and melena started 10 days after septic episode. A: following renograffin injection dye is seen accumulating in gastric lumen (large dye filled area on left). B: late film showing dye collected along greater curvature of stomach. C: repeat injection 30 minutes after start of pitressin infusion. The left gastric artery is no longer visualized and no further extravasation of dye is seen, indicating that bleeding has been controlled. The patient made a complete recovery without the need for surgical intervention.

is appropriately constricted, pitressin infusion is then started at 0.2 units per min in 5% dextrose at 0.5-1.0 ml per min. If the patient's condition permits, a further dye injection should be carried out one half to 1 hour later to ascertain that bleeding has indeed been arrested (Figure 5-1). If necessary, the infusion rate may be increased to 0.4 units per min. Once hemorrhage has been controlled for 12 to 24 hours, the infusion rate may be gradually tapered over the next 24 to 36 hours as long as the situation remains stable. After cessation of pitressin infusion, the catheter is left in place for a further 24 hours and perfused with dextrose solution. If bleeding does not recur, the catheter is then removed. Patients with bleeding duodenal ulcer present a special problem, since continued perfusion may result in necrosis of the duodenum. Therefore, this technique is usually utilized only to allow for adequate preparation of the patient for operation. Mention has already been made of the increased mortality of operation in patients with portal hypertension and hemorrhage from a source other than esophageal varices. It may be that this population of patients should be studied with a view to determining the efficacy of prolonged infusion in this circumstance.

Hemorrhage from the lower esophagus, whether secondary to esophagitis or the Mallory-Weiss tear, can usually be controlled by infusion of the left gastric artery. Bleeding from a gastric ulcer may be controlled with pitressin infusion into the left gastric artery as well, although autologous clot injected superselectively has also been utilized in this situation (87). Before using autologous clot, one must document the entire circulation in question. Further, in dog experiments (88) both pre- and post-emboli vasoconstrictors were needed to prevent clot fragmentation. However, in view of the generally good results with surgical treatment of bleeding peptic ulcer, use of these new modalities of therapy must be more fully proved before their general use can be recommended.

Hemorrhage from lesions of the large bowel usually responds to pitressin infusion of the appropriate vessel, that is the inferior mesenteric artery for rectum, descending colon, splenic flexure, and distal transverse colon and the superior mesenteric artery for the colon proximal to these areas. It must be remembered that collateral circulation is extensive, and it may be necessary to infuse both arteries in patients with transverse colon lesions.

OPERATIVE TRATMENT IN GASTROINTESTINAL HEMORRHAGE: A SURGEON'S VIEWPOINT

Duodenal ulcer.   A multiplicity of operations is available for the treatment of peptic ulcer disease. These operations include vagotomy and drainage procedure (pyloroplasties or gastrojejunostomy), subtotal gastrectomy, vagotomy and antrectomy and, more recently, parietal cell vagectomy. In a patient with bleeding duodenal ulcer the surgeon must strive to perform the most effective operation in terms of control of bleeding and prevention of recurrence of ulcer disease. This must be balanced against morbidity and mortality associated with the procedure. In the elective situation, parietal cell vagectomy without drainage will probably have least morbidity and mortality, while vagotomy and antrectomy will probably have the least recurrence rate. Unfortunately, the former procedure is inadequate for control of bleeding unless the duodenum is opened and the ulcer suture ligated. Furthermore, this would be more time-consuming than truncal vagectomy with drainage. Vagotomy and antrectomy, on the other hand, will afford greatest control of bleeding and protection from recurrence, but at the cost of increased morbidity from duodenal stump or anastomotic leakage. Subtotal gastrectomy has been shown to be associated with high mortality (as high as 30% in one series) when it is used in the emergency treatment for bleeding duodenal ulcer. Because of these considerations and on the basis of data from several studies, vagotomy and pyloroplasty with suture ligation of the bleeding ulcer appears to be the best procedure, even though the rebleeding rate in the immediate postoperative period may be higher than after either of the resective procedures. One should not, however, adopt a rigid attitude toward the performance of one procedure to the exclusion of the others. A more rational approach would be the performance of the best possible operation which circumstances dictate in that patient, such as age of the patient, cardiovascular and other associated disorders, intraoperative hemodynamic status of the patient, nutritional status, and technical considerations, as well as the surgeon's own experience with any of the available procedures. Thus in the patient with unstable cardiovascular status who has received much blood and whose duodenum is difficult to dissect, vagotomy, pyloroplasty, and suture ligation of the ulcer would seem most appropriate. On the other hand, the more stable patient with a long history of severe ulcer diathesis would be better treated with vagotomy and antrectomy depending on technical considerations.

Gastric ulcer.   There is little doubt that bleeding from a chronic gastric ulcer, unassociated with duodenal ulcer, is best controlled by subtotal gastric resection, especially when there is active bleeding. Such operative treatment will also allow excision of an unrecognized malignancy in the ulcer. If the location of the ulcer is such that a local resection of the ulcer alone is feasible, then this should be the preferred procedure in the poor risk patient. Unfortunately, gastric ulcers are not infrequently located high in the stomach in relatively inaccessible areas for resectional therapy. Under these circumstances, suture ligation of the ulcer from inside the stomach, or ligation of the feeding vessel (frequently the left gastric artery) from outside the stomach, combined with vagectomy and a drainage procedure, or antrectomy should be considered.

If gastric ulceration is associated with duodenal ulcer disease, then excisional therapy alone is not sufficient without control of gastric acid hypersecretion, and such ulcerations should be treated in the same manner as bleeding duodenal ulcers.

Erosive gastritis and stress ulceration.   Controversy continues to abound regarding surgical treatment of gastritis and erosions. Many patients with these disorders have other associated diseases, such as alcoholism, sepsis, burns, and intracranial pathology. Ideally then, the most expeditious operation with the least complication rate would be preferred. Unfortunately, such operations as vagotomy, pyloroplasty, and suture ligation of bleeding points have been followed by prohibitive rebleeding rates in most series (38,39,40). Near-total or total gastrectomy, on the other hand, are almost always effective for control of bleeding, but the associated morbidity and mortality rates are high. Thus, once again, the surgeon must resolve this dilemma by "tailoring" his operation to the preoperative and intraoperative circumstances. More specifically, in the younger patient without preexisting cardiovascular disease, the "lesser" procedure of vagotomy, drainage, and suture ligation of bleeding points should be considered. In this way, the patient is spared the long-term metabolic impairments of near-total or total gastrectomy. The surgeon, however, must be prepared to perform the latter procedures if bleeding continues or recurs. On the other hand, the older patient with marginal cardiovascular reserve cannot be allowed the added insult of hemodynamic instability from continued or recurrent hemorrhage, and aggressive surgical treatment is warranted in such patients. Under these circumstances, a higher complication rate and mortality is to be expected, but in the current era of better management of shock, sepsis, and cardiopulmonary failure, one would hope for improved survival rates. Nonetheless, since surgical treatment for this problem is very difficult and often hazardous, every effort must be made to avoid the need for surgical intervention. Intraarterial pitressin infusion may offer one alternative. Another is intensive antacid therapy, which has recently been claimed to be effective in arresting bleeding in 89% of 49 patients in this category.

Bleeding esophageal varices.   No other intraabdominal procedure taxes the surgeon's ingenuity and skill more than operation for control of bleeding esophageal varices. Not only are portal decompressive operations difficult, but there is always the imminent danger of uncontrollable bleeding from dilated, frail intra-abdominal veins, as well as continuous blood loss because of poor clotting function. It is thus apparent that the surgeon treating such patients should be experienced in the performance of the various portal decompressive procedures. Rapidity of operation (and, hence, reduced anesthetic time), minimal blood loss to avoid shock (thus minimizing further impairment of hepatic hemodynamics), and a technically satisfactory shunt, which will not thrombose, are prerequisites to the survival of such patients.

Of all the portal decompressive operations, the portacaval shunts (end-to-side or side-to-side) have alone stood the test of time as effective in the long-term control of variceal hemorrhage (43,44,51,52). The end-to-side shunt is easier to perform and probably is attended by a lower incidence of encephalopathy, than is the side-to-side shunt. This is because the latter shunt may divert a greater amount of portal blood from the liver due to reversal of flow in the hepatic limb of the portal vein after anastomosis. For the same reason, however, the side-to-side portacaval shunt is more effective in the control of ascites, because of better decompression of the hepatic vascular bed. Thus this shunt should be considered in patients with ascites.

The mesocaval shunt (90), using an interposed large-bore prosthetic vascular graft, has been advocated as an excellent alternative to the portacaval shunts. It should be remembered, however, that this is effectively a side-to-side shunt and would be expected to be attended with a similar incidence of post-shunt encephalopathy, although its proponents believe the incidence to be less. Aside from these considerations, the mesocaval interposition shunt, for surgeons not experienced in performance of the standard portacaval shunts, is an easier operation. Furthermore, it is the best alternative when the portal vein is thrombosed, or there has been a previous right upper quadrant operation making dissection more difficult.

The standard proximal splenorenal shunt has very little to offer in the emergency situation. Its thrombosis rate is higher in most hands, and it is a technically more demanding operation. The distal selective splenorenal shunt (91) has great potential in elective situations, because of minimal deprivation of blood flow from the liver and, hence, potentially a reduced incidence of post-shunt encephalopathy. Nonetheless, in the actively bleeding patient because this operation is more time-consuming, and also theoretically not as rapidly effective in lowering portal pressure as portacaval shunts, it should probably not be used for the control of variceal hemorrhage.

Even in experienced hands, the mortality following portal decompression in emergency situations can be as high as 40% to 60%, even in patients who are acceptable operative candidates. But these are tolerable figures when one considers the alternative of a 100% mortality if bleeding is uncontrolled by other means (see Chapter 5). We believe, therefore, that no patient with uncontrollable bleeding from varices should be refused operation. With a team approach, including gastroenterologist, anesthesiologist, angiographer, and a surgeon interested and experienced in treatment of portal hypertension, the mortality figures should be lowered considerably.

Massive hemorrhage from diverticular disease of the colon.   Surgical intervention is indicated when colonic hemorrhage due to diverticular disease cannot be controlled by angiographic or other nonoperative means. If the bleeding site has been localized by angiography, then colonic resection is the obvious solution. The extent of resection should be dictated by the extent of diverticulosis. Thus, if at operation diverticula are limited to the right colon, then right hemicolectomy is the operation of choice. The choice of ileostomy and mucous fistula, as against primary anastomosis, must be determined by the surgeon at operation with consideration to fecal content of the bowel, vascular supply, and preoperative preparation. If, on the other hand, despite localization of bleeding to one area, there is universal diverticulosis, technical considerations as well as concern for recurrent bleeding and future difficulties would, in my opinion, necessitate subtotal colectomy as the operative treatment of choice. Ileoproctostomy is followed by troublesome diarrhea in some patients. However, since this problem can usually be managed satisfactorily, it should not be a deterrent to the use of this operation, when it is indicated. When the colonic bleeding site has not been located preoperatively, subtotal colectomy should be considered also, since studies have shown that bleeding from right-sided colonic diverticular disease is as frequent, if not more frequent, than from the left side. However, the extent of colonic resection must be determined on the extent of the diverticular disease and, if possible, by intraoperative localization of the bleeding site, using endoscopy or dye studies. Once again, the same considerations should be given regarding primary versus delayed anastomosis.

Not infrequently, the cause of colonic bleeding remains obscure even with the abdomen opened. If obvious diverticulosis or other colonic lesions are not found, then consideration should be given to the performance of intraoperative angiography. The right and middle colic and the inferior mesenteric arteries can be cannulated with a small scalp-vein needle and contrast material can then be injected. The surgeon may be rewarded by extravasation of dye indicating the source of bleeding.

REFERENCES

1. Tibbs, D. J.: Blood volume in gastro-intestinal hemorrhage. *Lancet,* **2:**266, 1956.
2. Tudhope, G. R.: The loss and replacement of red cells in patients with acute gastro-intestinal hemorrhage. *Quart. J. Med.,* **27:**543, 1958.
3. Ebert, R. V., Stead, E. A., and Gibson, J. G.: Response of normal subjects to acute blood loss, with special reference to the mechanism of restoration of blood volume. *Arch. Intern. Med.* **68:**578, 1941.
4. Jones, F. A., and Gummer, J. W. P.: *Clinical Gastroenterology.* Blackwell, Oxford, 1960.
5. Hellers, G., and Imre, T.: Impact of change to early diagnosis and surgery in major upper gastro-intestinal bleeding. *Lancet,* **2:**1250, 1975.
6. Jones, F. A.: Modern Trends in Gastroenterology. Butterworth and Co., Ltd. London, 1952.
7. Dawson, A. M: Intragastric milk drip in the treatment of upper gastro-intestinal hemorrhage. *Lancet,* **1:**73, 1956.
8. Chandler, G. N., and Watkinson, G.: Gastric aspiration in hematemesis. *Lancet,* **2:**1170, 1953.
9. Schiller, K. F. R., Truelove, S. C., and Williams, G. D.: Hematemesis and melena, with special reference to factors influencing outcome. *Brit. Med. J.* **2:**7, 1970.
10. McHorse, T. S., Williamson, G. R., Johnson, R. F., and Schenker, S.: Effect of acute viral hepatitis in man on the disposition and elimination of meperidine. *Gastroenterology,* **68:**775, 1975.
11. Klotz, U., Avent, G. R., Hoyumpa, A., Schenker, S., and Wilkinson, G. R.: The effects of age and liver disease on the disposition and elimination of diazepam in adult man. *J. Clin. Invest.* **55:**347, 1975.
12. Lieber, C. S.: Hepatic and metabolic effects of alcohol (1966 to 1973). *Gastroenterology,* **65:** 821, 1973.
13. Jones, F. A.: Hematemesis and melena: With speical reference to causation and to the factors influencing the mortality from bleeding peptic ulcers. *Gastroenterology,* **30:**166, 1956.
14. Palmer, E. D.: The vigorous diagnostic approach to upper gastrointestinal tract hemorrhage. A 23-year prospective study of 1400 cases. *JAMA,* **207:**1477, 1969.
15. Cotton, P. B., Rosenberg, M. T., Waldram, R. P. W., and Axon, A. T. R.: Early endoscopy of esophagus, stomach and duodenal bulb in patients with hematemesis and melena. *Brit. Med J.,* **2:**505, 1973.
16. Schiff, L., Stevens, R. J., Shapiro, N., and Goodman, S.: Observations on oral administration of citrated blood in man—Effect on stools. *Amer. J. Med. Sci.* **203:**409, 1942.
17. Kalm, R. M., and Smith, F. W.: Panendoscopy in the early diagnosis of upper gastrointestinal bleeding. *Gastroenterology,* **65:**728, 1973.
18. Sandlow, L. J., Beeker, G. H., Spellberg, M. A., Allen, H. A., Berg, M., Berry, L. H., and Newman, E. A.: A prospective randomized study of the management of UGI hemorrhage. *Amer. J. Gastro.* **61:**282, 1974.
19. Morris, D. W., Levine, G. M., Soloway, R. D., Miller, W. T., Marin, G. A.: Prospective randomized study of diagnosis and outcome in acute upper gastro-intestinal bleeding: Endoscopy versus conventional radiography. *Amer. J. Digest. Dis.* **20:**1103, 1975.

20. Gordon-Taylor, G.: Present position of surgery in the treatment of bleeding peptic ulcer. *Brit. J. Surg.* **33:**336, 1946.

21. Finsterer, H.: Operative treatment of severe gastric hemorrhage of ulcer origin. *Lancet,* **2:**303, 1936.

22. Lewin, D. C., and Truelove, S.: Hematemesis with special reference to chronic peptic ulcer. *Brit. Med. J.* **1:**383, 1949.

23. Northfield, T. C.: Factors predisposing to recurrent hemorrhage after acute gastrointestinal bleeding. *Brit. Med. J.* **1:**26, 1971.

24. Carruthers, R. K., Giles, G. R., Clark, C. G., and Goligher, J. C.: Conservative surgery for bleeding peptic ulcer. *Brit. Med. J.* **1:**80, 1967.

25. Farris, J. M., and Smith, G. K.: Appraisal of long-term results after vagotomy and pyloroplasty in 100 patients with bleeding duodenal ulcer. *Ann. Surg.* **166:**630, 1967.

26. Balint, J. A., Cooper, G. W., Price, E. C. V., Pulvertaft, C. N., and Swynnerton, B. F.: The management of anastomotic ulceration. *Lancet,* **2:**551, 1957.

27. Richardson, C. T., and Walsh, J. H.: Histamine H_2—Receptor antagonist in Zollinger-Ellison syndrome. *New England J. Med.* **294:**133, 1976.

28. Balint, J. A., and Spence, M. P.: Pyloric stenosis—A review of 118 consecutive cases. *Brit. Med. J.* **1:**890, 1959.

29. Curling, T. B.: An acute ulceration of the duodenum in cases of burns. *Med. Chir. Trans.* London, **25:**260, 1842.

30. Stillman, J. J., and Silen, W.: Stress ulcers. *Lancet,* **2:**1303, 1972.

31. Cushing, H.: Peptic ulcers and the brain. *Surg. Gynec. and Obstet.* **55:**1, 1932.

32. Davenport, H. W.: Back diffusion of acid through the gastric mucosa and its physiological consequences. In Progress in *Gastroenterology,* Vol. II, G. B. J. Glass (ed), Grune & Stratton, New York, 1970.

33. Stillman, J. J., Bushnell, L. S., Goldman, H., and W. Silen: Respiratory failure, hypotension, sepsis and jaundice—a clinical syndrome associated with lethal hemorrhage from acute stress ulceration. *Amer. J. Surg.* **117:**523, 1969.

34. Beil, A. B., Mannix, H., and Beal, J. M.: Massive upper gastrointestinal hemorrhage after operation. *Amer. J. Surg.* **108:**324, 1964.

35. Harkins, H. N.: Acute ulcer of the duodenum (Curling's ulcer) as a complication of burns, relation to sepsis. *Surgery,* 1939.

36. Mears, F. B.: Autopsy survey of peptic ulcer associated with other disease. *Surgery,* **34:**640, 1953.

37. Silen, W., and Skillman, J. J.: Stress ulcer, acute erosive gastritis and the gastric mucosal barrier. *Adv. Intern. Med.* **19:**195, 1974.

38. Menguy, R., Gadacz, T., and Zatchuk, R.: The surgical management of acute gastric mucosal bleeding. *Arch. Surg.* **99:**198, 1969.

39. Luke, D. J., and Dragstedt, L. R.: Massive bleeeding due to acute hemorrhagic gastritis. *Arch. Surg.,* **101:**550, 1970.

40. Desmond, A. M., and Reynolds, K. W.: Erosive gastritis: Its diagnosis, management and surgical treatment. *Brit. J. Surg.* **59:**5, 1972.

41. Athanasoulis, C. A., Baum, S., Waltman, A. C., Ring, E. J., Imbembo, A., and Vander Salm, T. J.: Intraarterial posterior pituitary extract for acute gastric mucosal hemorrhage. *New England J. Med.* **290:**597, 1974.

42. Brick, I. B., and Palmer, E. D.: One thousand cases of portal cirrhosis of the liver. *Arch. Intern. Med.* **113:**501, 1964.
43. Orloff, M. J.: Emergency portacaval shunt: A comparative study of shunt, varix ligation and nonsurgical treatment of bleeding esophageal varices in unselected patients with cirrhosis. *Ann. Surg.* **166:**456, 1967.
44. Mikkelsen, W. P.: Therapeutic protacaval shunt: Preliminary data on controlled trial and morbid effects of acute hepatic necrosis. *Arch. Surg.* **106:**302, 1974.
45. Winkler, K.: Selection of patients with cirrhosis of the liver for shunt surgery. *Scand. J. Gastro.* **7:**679, 1972.
46. Mikkelsen, W. P.: Emergency portacaval shunt. *Rev. Surg.* **19:**141, 1962.
47. Baum, S., Athanasoulis, C. A., Waltman, A. C., and Rug, E. J.: Gastrointestinal hemorrhage, II. Angiographic diagnosis and control. *Adv. Surgery,* **7:**149, 1973.
48. George, P., Brown, C., Ridgway, G., Crofts, B., and Sherlock, S.: Emergency esophageal transection in uncontrolled variceal hemorrhage. *Brit. J. Surg.* **60:**635, 1973.
49. Conn, H. O.: Hazards attending the use of esophageal tamponade. *New England J. Med.* **259:**701, 1958.
50. Roberts, H. R., and Cederbaum, A. I.: The liver and blood coagulation: Physiology and pathology. *Gastroenterology,* **63:**297, 1972.
51. Jackson, F. C., Perrin, E. B., Felix, W. R., and Smith, A. G.: A clinical investigation of the portacaval shunt. V. Survival analysis of the therapeutic shunt. *Ann. Surg.* **174:**672, 1971.
52. Resnick, R. H., Iber, F. L., Ishihara, A. M., Chalmers, T. C., Zimmerman, H., and the Boston Interhospital Liver Group: A controlled study of the therapeutic portacaval shunt. *Gastroenterology,* **67:**843, 1974.
53. Conn, H. O., and Lindenmuth, W. W.: Prophylactic portacaval anastomosis in cirrhotic patients with esophageal varices. *New England J. Med.* **279:**725, 1968.
54. Resnick, R. H., Chalmers, T. C., Ishihara, A. M., Garceau, A. J., Callow, A. D., Schimmel, E. M., O'Hara, E. T., and the Boston Inter-hospital Liver Group: A controlled study of the prophylactic portacaval shunt. *Ann. Intern. Med.* **70:**675, 1969.
55. Saylor, J. L., and Tedesco, F. J.: Mallory-Weiss syndrome in perspective. *Amer. J. Digest. Dis.* In Press.
56. Baum, S., Alhanasoulis, C. A., and Waltman, A. C.: Angiographic diagnosis and control of large bowel bleeding. *Dis. Colon and Rectum,* **17:**447, 1974.
57. Rutherford, R. B., and Akers, D. R.: Meckel's diverticulum—A review of 148 pediatric patients with special reference to the pattern of bleeding and to meso-diverticular vascular bands. *Surgery,* **59:**615, 1966.
58. Rigg, B. M., and Ewing, M. R.: Current attitudes to diverticulitis with particular reference to colonic bleeding. *Arch. Surg.* **92:**321, 1961.
59. Bolt, D. E., and Hughes, L. E.: Diverticulitis: A follow-up of 100 cases. *Brit. Med. J.,* **1:**1205, 1966.
60. Broders, C. N.: Bleeding from diverticula of the colon. *Surg. Clin. North America,* **52:**315, 1972.

61. Manousos, O. N., Truelove, S. C., and Lumsden, K.: Prevalence of colonic diverticulosis in general population of Oxford area. *Brit. Med. J.* **2:**762, 1967.

62. Noer, R. J., Hamilton, J. E., Williams, D. J., and Broughton, D. S.: Rectal hemorrhage: Moderate and severe. *Ann. Surg.* **155:**794, 1962.

63. Edwards, F. C., and Truelove, S. C.: The course and prognosis of ulcerative colitis. *Gut,* **4:**299, 1973; **5:**1, 1974.

64. *Crohn's Disease.* Brooke, B. W. (ed), W. B. Saunders Co., London, Philadelphia, 1972.

65. McHardy, G., Bechtold, J. E., and McHardy, R. J.: Hemorrhage from primary disease of the mesenteric small intestine—Review of the literature and analysis of 216 cases. *Gastroenterology,* **28:**17, 1955.

66. Byrne, J. J., Guardione, V. A., and Williams, L. F.: Massive gastrointestinal hemorrhage. *Amer. J. Surg.* **120:**312, 1970.

67. Wirthlin, L. S., Van Urk, H., Malt, R. B., and Malt, R. A.: Predictors of surgical mortality in patients with cirrhosis and nonvariceal gastroduodenal bleeding. *Surg. Gyn. Ob.* **139:**65, 1974.

68. White, R. I., Harrington, D. P., Novak, G., Miller, F. J., Giorgeana, F. A., and Sheff, R. N.: Pharmacologic control of hemorrhagic gastritis. Clinical and experimental results. *Radiology,* **111:**549, 1974.

69. Johnson, W. C., and Widrich, W. C.: Efficacy of selective splanchnic arteriography and vasopressin perfusion in diagnosis and treatment of GI hemorrhage. *Amer. J. Surg.* **131:**481, 1976.

70. Novelline, R. A., Waltman, A. C., Athanasoulis, C. A., and Baum, S.: Recent advances in abdominal angiography. *Adv. Intern. Med.* **21:**417, 1976.

71. Athanasoulis, C. A., Waltman, A. C., Novelline, R. A., Phillips, D. A., and Baum, S.: Intraarterial infusions of vasopressin for the control of upper gastrointestinal hemorrhage. In *Gastrointestinal Emergencies* (Clearfield & Denosa, ed.); the 34th Hahnemann Symposium, Grune & Stratton, 1976, p. 37.

72. Athanasoulis, C. A., Waltman, A. C., Imbemba, A. L., Coureg, W. R., and Baum, S.: Control of hemorrhagic gastritis by intra-arterial infusion of vasopressin. *Gastroenterology,* **64:**693, 1973.

73. Conn, H. O., Ramsby, G. R., and Storer, E. H.: Selective intraarterial vasopressin in the treatment of upper gastrointestinal hemorrhage. *Gastroenterology,* **63:**634, 1972.

74. King, E. J., Baum, S., Athanasoulis, C., and Waltman, A. C.: Angiography in the diagnosis and treatment of nonvariceal bleeding in patients with portal hypertension. *Surg. Gyn. Ob.* **139:**205, 1974.

75. Athanasoulis, C. A., Brown, B., and Shapiro, J. H.: Angiography in the diagnosis and management of bleeding stress ulcers and gastritis. *Amer. J. Surg.* **125:**468, 1973.

76. Conn, H. O., Ramsby, G. R., Storer, E. H., Hutchnick, M. G., Joski, P. H., Phillips, M. M., Cohen, G. A., Fields, G. N., and Petroski, N.: Intra-arterial vasopressin in the treatment of upper gastrointestinal hemorrhage: A prospective controlled clinical trial. *Gastroenterology,* **68:**211, 1975.

77. Eisenberg, H., Laufer, I., and Skittman, J. J.: Arteriographic diagnosis and management of suspected colonic diverticular hemorrhage. *Gastroenterology,* **64:**1091, 1973.

78. Baum, S., Rosch, J., Dotter, C. T., and King, E. J.: Selective mesenteric

arterial infusions in the management of massive diverticular hemorrhage. *New England J. Med.* **288:**1269, 1973.

79. Rosch, J., Dotter, C. T., and Antonovic, R.: Selective vasoconstrictor infusion in the management of arterio-capillary gastro-intestinal hemorrhage. *Amer. J. Roent. Rad. Ther. & Nuc. Med.* **116:**279, 1972.

80. Nusbaum, M., Baum, S., Kuroda, K., and Balkemore, W.: Control of portal hypertension by selective mesenteric arterial drug infusion. *Arch. Surg.* **97:**1003, 1968.

81. Winawer, S. J., Sherlock, P., Sonenberg, P., and Vanamer, P.: Control of stress ulcer hemorrhage with human growth hormone. *Gastroenterology,* **64:**853, 1973.

82. Nusbaum, M., Baum, S., Blakemore, W. S., and Tumen, H.: Clinical experience with selective intra-arterial infusion of vasopressin in the control of gastro-intestinal bleeding from arterial sources. *Amer. J. Surg.* **123:**165, 1972.

83. Lauson, H. R., and Bacanegra, M.: Clearance of exogenous vasopressin from plasma of dogs. *Amer. J. Phys.* **200:**493, 1961.

84. Rosch, J., Dotter, C. T., and Rose, R. W.: Selective arterial infusions of vasoconstrictors in acute gastrointestinal bleeding. *Radiology,* **99:**27, 1971.

85. Athanasoulis, C. A., Baum, S., Waltman, A. C., King, E. J., Imbemba, A., and Salm, T. J. V.: Control of acute gastric mucosal hemorrhage. *New England J. Med.* **290:**597, 1974.

86. Marubbio, A. T., Lombardo, R. P., and Holt, P. R.: Control of variceal bleeding by superior mesenteric artery pitressin infusions—complications and indications. *Amer. J. Digest. Dis.* **18:**539, 1973.

87. Prochaska, J. M., Fuge, M. W., and Johnstrude, I. S.: Left gastric artery embolisation for control of gastric bleeding: A complication. *Radiology,* **107:**521, 1973.

88. Rosch, J., Dotter, C. T., and Brown, M. J.: Selective arterial embolisation. *Radiology,* **102:**303, 1972.

89. Simonian, S. J., and Curtis, L. E.: Treatment of hemorrhagic gastritis by antacid. *Ann. Surg.* **184:**429, 1976.

90. Drapanas, T.: Interposition mesocaval shunt for treatment of portal hypertension. *Ann. Surg.* **176:**435, 1972.

91. Warren, D. W., Zeppa, R., and Fomon, J. J.: Selective transsplenic decompression of gastroesophageal varices by distal splenorenal shunt. *Ann. Surg.* **166:**437, 1967.

6

GASTROINTESTINAL HEMORRHAGE OF UNKNOWN ORIGIN

Recurrent episodes of bleeding from the gastrointestinal tract without a firm diagnosis as to source present a disturbing problem for the patient and the physician. Few studies have been directed to this specific problem. For the purpose of this discussion, bleeding of unknown site is defined as documented bleeding in a patient in whom no source of bleeding has been found after full clinical, hematologic, radiologic, and upper and lower intestinal endoscopic investigation, not necessarily including angiography. The prevalence of this problem is very difficult to determine. Birke and Engstedt (1) reviewed the experience at the Karolinska Hospital in Stockholm from 1941 to 1951. The patients in their study conformed to the definition given above, except that no endoscopy was performed. Of 1252 patients with bleeding, a firm diagnosis as to source was not made in 191, that is 15%. Douvres and Glass (2) in a series of 800 patients in whom endoscopy was regularly employed found that 15.5% remained unexplained. Similar findings were also reported by Hirschowitz and co-workers (3) from a study of the value of fiberoptic gastroscopy in the investigation of patients with upper gastrointestinal bleeding.

In approaching the question of how actively to investigate such patients, it is helpful to have some information as to the likely long-term course of such cases. Birke and Engstedt followed their 191 patients for 4 to 14 years following their entry into the study (1). Eighty-six (45%) of their patients never bled again and remained classified as cryptogenic bleeders. Eighty-eight (46%) ultimately had a diagnosis established because of recurrent problems. The diagnoses included peptic ulcer (49 patients), benign tumors (6 patients), malignant tumors (24 patients), and other diagnoses (9 patients). The 24 patients with malignant tumors included 7 cases each of gastric and pancreatic cancer, 5 with carcinoma of the colon and 3 with carcinoma of the ampulla of Vater. Since many of these lesions would be diagnosable by endoscopy, it would be reasonable to assume that this investigative procedure would reduce the number of undiagnosed cases. The fact that others using endoscopy had a similar incidence of cryptogenic cases (2, 3) suggests that some of the lesions found by Birke and Engstedt (1) in follow-up were not the source of the initial bleeds. Douvres and Glass (2) reported that one third of their undiagnosed cases returned with recurrent hemorrhage. They indicated that in many of these cases a diagnosis as to the source of bleeding was made at the second admission. In patients presenting with melena only, as contrasted to those with hematemesis, the frequency of an undiagnosed source of bleeding is much higher, ranging from 27 to 43% in various series (2).

The most common sources of bleeding that present difficulties in diagnosis are listed in Table 6-1. Small-bowel lesions account for about 2% of major gastrointestinal hemorrhages (4) and are a frequent cause of cryptogenic bleeding, since this area of the digestive tract is not readily accessible to endoscopic evaluation, and radiology of the small bowel presents technical problems because of overlapping loops of bowel. McHardy et al (4), based on a study on 216 cases of small-bowel disease, found that 25% presented with hemorrhage, and that 38% of these had pain associated with the bleeding episode. In about one half the patients the presentation is with melena and in the rest with red blood per rectum. Two thirds of these patients also gave a history of previous bleeding or

Table 6-1
Potential Causes of Bleeding of Obscure Source

Disease	Cardinal Features	Diagnosis
Meckel's diverticulum	Usually reddish blood with pain; < 25 years	Pertechnitate scan Angiography during bleed
Small-bowel tumors	Recurrent anemia Melena or red blood > 25 years	Repeated SBFT* Angiography; string test
Vascular lesions		
A-V aneurysm	Recurrent painless	Angiography
Telengiectasia	bleeds; may have	Telengiectasia by PE
Angiodysplasia	mucocutaneous lesions	or endoscopy
Cardiovascular		
Aortic Stenosis††	Recurrent hemorrhage with aortic stenosis	Angiography
ASHD††●	Recurrent hemorrhage	Angiography
Hematologic disorders		
Lymphoma	Usually asymptomatic bleeding; may have pain	Radiologic, endoscopic
Clotting disorders	Bleeding tendency	Clotting tests
Hereditary disorders		
Pseudoxanthoma elasticum	Family history; cutaneous lesions (Table 2-2)	Clinical
Ehlers-Danlos	Perioral pigmentation	Clinical
Peutz-Jeghers		Clinical and radiologic

* SBFT = small-bowel follow-through examination.
● ASHD = arteriosclerotic heart disease.
†† Most commonly found to have angiodysplasia.

anemia (4). Thus this clinical history and presentation, in patients with few physical findings, should raise a strong suspicion of small-bowel disease. Recent advances in understanding the hormonal control of intestinal motility hold out the promise of improved radiologic examination of the small bowel and should, therefore, improve diagnostic accuracy. Cholecystokinin can be used to accelerate intestinal propulsion of barium, while secretin will arrest it. Thus fluoroscopy of the small bowel could be accomplished in a much shorter time. When a suspicious area is seen, motility can be arrested with secretin, the area can be examined, and radiographs obtained. Another injection of cholecystokinin can then be given to restart motility. This technique still awaits full clinical evaluation. Even with this procedure, however, a Meckel's diverticulum may not be visualized. Although small-bowel tumors are a more likely cause of bleeding in older patients, Meckel's diverticulum must be considered in this clinical context in patients under the age of 25, especially if red blood is passed per rectum, since only 7% of these patients have melena (5). Technitium[99] pertechnitate scans can be used to identify ectopic gastric mucosa in a Meckel's diverticulum (6), since the pertechnitate ion is excreted by this mucosa in the same way as choloride ion. An example of a positve pertechnitate scan is shown in Figure 6-1. Isotope is seen concentrated in the lower abdomen in a young man presenting with bright red rectal bleeding. Since bleeding from a Meckel's diverticulum only occurs when ectopic gastric mucosa is present, isotopic imaging promises to be a very useful diagnostic modality in such patients.

Vascular lesions of the gastrointestinal tract are now more readily recognized because of the availability of selective angiography (7). Diagnosis by angiography is relatively easy during a bleeding episode, when extravasation of dye into the lumen is demonstrable. However, vascular malformations may be demonstrable even when not bleeding, and should be looked for in patients who have a recurrent bleeding episode after a previous cryptogenic hemorrhage. Since angiography is expensive, uncomfortable, and has some risk, and since many patients with one bleeding episode will either have no recurrences, or will have a diagnosis established by more routine measures in the future, we do not recommend angiography of all patients during the first episode. Clearly, as discussed in Chapter 5, if the bleeding is continuing, angiography may need to be undertaken for diagnostic or therapeutic reasons on an emergency basis. Usually selective arteriography should be performed in patients who remain a diagnostic problem after a second bleeding episode has been evaluated by routine methods. There has been much discussion in the literature about the incidence of obscure gastrointestinal bleeding in patients with aortic stenosis and arteriosclerotic heart disease. Douvres and Glass (2) reviewed this literature and found the evidence contradictory, with some series indicating an increased incidence of such bleeding in patients with aortic stenosis and others unable to confirm this. Since then, a study of 610 cases of valvular heart disease found seven instances of unexplained hemorrhage among 275 patients with aortic stenosis, but none among 335 patients with other valve involvement (8). The question, therefore, remains unanswered. In 3 patients with aortic stenosis and hemorrhage, selective angiography revealed submucosal vascular anomalies in the right colon (9). This observation is in line with the findings of Baum and colleagues, suggesting that angiodysplasia is more common in older patients with

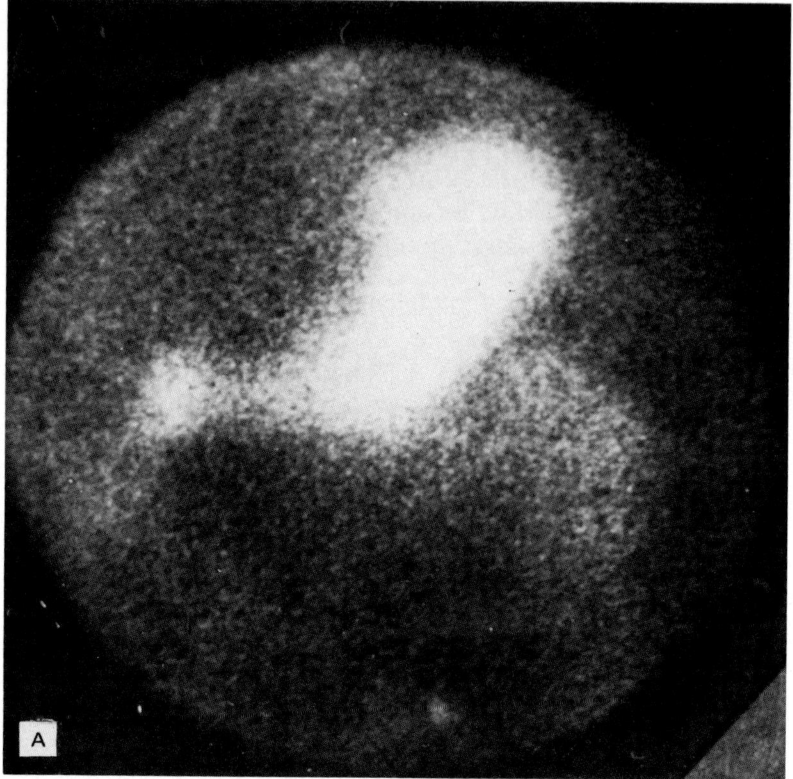

FIGURE 6-1

Pertechnitate scan to show Meckel's diverticulum. A: shows isotopic
outline of the stomach. B: shows accumulation of pertechnitate in right
lower quadrant (arrow) in Meckel's diverticulum. These studies were
obtained in a 22-year-old man with a history of excess alcohol ingestion,
and dark red rectal bleeding. UGI endoscopy was negative. The diagnosis
was confirmed at the time of surgical removal of the diverticulum.

arteriosclerotic heart disease (10). Mention should also be made of the collagen
vascular disorders such as Henoch-Schoenlein purpura, polyarteritis nodosa,
and systemic lupus erythematosus. These diseases are not uncommonly complicated by intestinal bleding, but it is rare for this to be the sole presenting symptom. Such patients commonly have associated abdominal pain, evidence of renal
disease, arthritis, or pulmonary lesions.

The hereditary syndromes associated with gastrointestinal bleeding are all
readily diagnosable on clinical grounds as discussed in Chapter 2. Careful family
history, examination of the skin, eyes, and buccal mucosa will reveal the typical
features of these disorders in almost every case. Therefore, the importance of a
complete clinical examination in all patients with bleeding cannot be overem-
phasized. Even though one of these diagnoses has been established, a complete
investigation of the gastrointestinal tract must be carried out when the patient is
first seen to exclude other more common causes of bleeding. Once it has been
established that no other lesion is present, these studies need not be repeated in

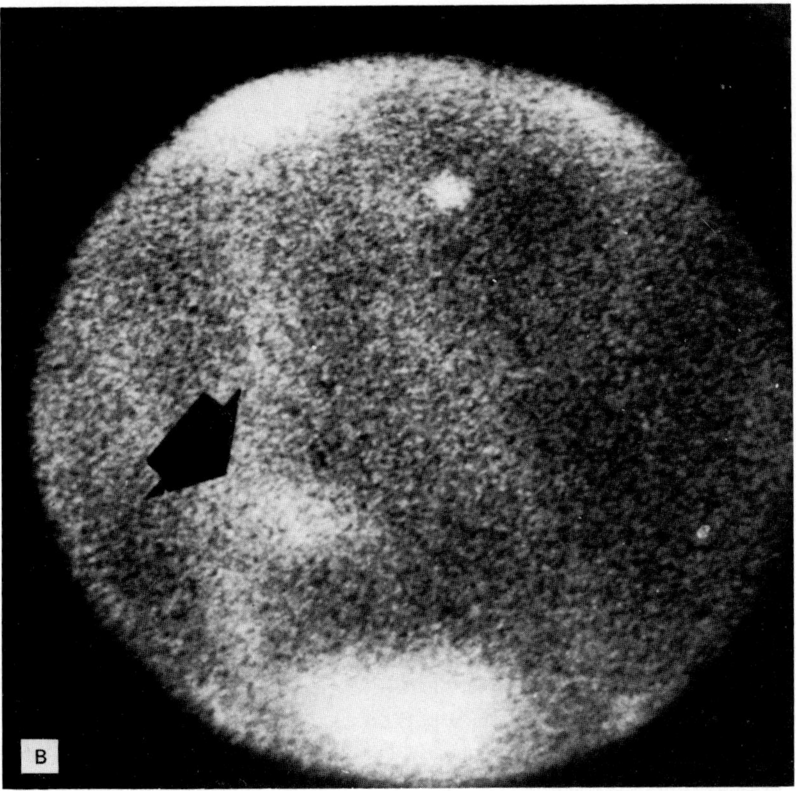

subsequent episodes, unless a change in the clinical presentation suggests development of another condition. Similar considerations apply to patients with acquired or inherited disorders of coagulation. Coagulation defects must be ruled out in all patients with bleeding by the studies outlined in Chapter 2 and Table 2-4. If a coagulation defect is detected, this must be corrected if possible, before a complete endoscopic evaluation is carried out.

What should be done with the patient who, after full clinical, hematologic, radiologic, and endoscopic evaluation, remains without a diagnosis as to the source of bleeding? There appear to be two courses of action open to the physician. If the bleeding has stopped, he is probably justified in taking a conservative course, since the experience of others has indicated that the majority of such patients will either have no further problem, or will be found to have a benign disorder that can be diagnosed and treated next time around (1,2). Of concern will be the 25% of patients reported by Birke and Engstedt (1), who later presented with malignant tumors and in whom the prognosis may have been made worse by the delay in diagnosis. We presently lack data to support or negate this possibility. The main reason for recommending the conservative approach to these patients is that, short of laparotomy, the tests available to try to localize the site of bleeding all depend on continuing bleeding, even if only occult. Laparotomy for obscure bleeding is generally rewarded by only a very low yield (2). The other alternative is presented by the patient who continues to have low-grade or occult bleeding. In these patients a number of procedures are available to aid in localizing the site of hemorrhage. Quantitative data on the value of these tests, however, are lacking. Douvres and Glass (2) have reviewed these procedures. Basically all are variations of the original Einhorn string test. These tests are most helpful when bleeding is slow (< 1 ml/min) or occult, since with more rapid blood loss localization becomes inaccurate due to spread of blood up and down the bowel. The original modification of this test was the use of intravenous fluorescein. The tape with lead markers, 5 cm apart, is passed into the small bowel as far as possible. The number of marks beyond the pylorus is noted on a plain film of the abdomen. Fluorescein is then injected intravenously and the tape is left in place for 5 to 10 minutes, and is then withdrawn. It is then inspected under an ultraviolet light and the point of fluorescence, if any, is noted and correlated with the film to judge the site of bleeding. More recently, this test has been modified by using Cr^{51} labeled autologous red blood cells, and passing the tape over a Geiger counter. Others have used Cr^{51} labeled red cells after passage of a long intestinal tube (Miller-Abbott or Kantor tube). Serial aspirations of intestinal content are then made during withdrawal of the tube under radiological control. This method can also be used to quantitate blood loss (11). Douvres and Glass claim to have had good success with this procedure (2). However, the data available are only anecdotal. If these procedures fail to localize the bleeding site, and bleeding is still continuing at a significant rate requiring replacement therapy by transfusion, the question of laparotomy must be reconsidered. Before surgery is undertaken, a very careful review of all medications taken by the patient should again be done to rule out the possibility of drug-induced hemorrhage. If this is again negative, repeat endoscopy and angiography may be helpful. If by this time the bleeding still continues, laparotomy will probably be necessary. The yield of convincing positive diagnoses is likely to be less than 30% after exploration.

If the bleeding has either stopped or slowed to the point where oral iron therapy is sufficient to maintain normal hemoglobin levels, it is often best to continue careful observation of the patient while under conservative management. If any change in the patient's clinical picture develops during this period, reinvestigation and, if appropriate, more aggressive therapy can be instituted. This approach avoids subjecting the patient to the hazards of unnecessary invasive diagnostic procedures and surgery. The practice of "blind subtotal gastrectomy," which was popular at one time in the hope of curing these patients, has been proved to be not only unrewarding but unacceptable because of the complications following gastric resection in 10% to 20% of patients.

REFERENCES

1. Birke, G., and Engstedt, L.: Melena and Hematemesis—A follow-up investigation with special reference to bleeding of unknown origin. *Gastroenterologia*, **85:**97, 1956.
2. Douvres, P. A., and Glass, G. B. J.: Cryptogenic gastrointestinal bleeding. In *Progress in Gastroenterology*, Vol. II, G. B. J. Glass (ed), Grune and Stratton, New York and London, 1970.

3. Hirschowitz, B. I., Luketic, G. C., Balint, J. A., and Fulton, W. F.: Early fiberscope endoscopy for upper gastrointestinal bleeding. *Amer. J. Digest. Dis.* **8:**816, 1963.

4. McHardy, G., Bechtold, J. E., and McHardy, R. J.: Hemorrhage from primary disease of the mesenteric small intestine—Review of the literature and analysis of 216 cases. *Gastroenterology,* **28:**17, 1955.

5. Rutherford, R. B., Akers, D. R.: Meckel's diverticulum—A review of 148 patients with special reference to the pattern of bleeding and to mesodiverticular vascular bands. *Surgery,* **59:**618, 1966.

6. Eisenberg, D., and Sherwood, C. E.: Bleeding Meckel's diverticulum diagnosed by enteroscopy and radioisotope imaging. *Amer. J. Digest. Dis.* **20:**573, 1975.

7. Baum, S., Athanasoulis, C. A., Waltman, A. C., and Rug, E. J.: Gastrointestinal hemorrhage, II. Angiographic diagnosis and control. *Adv. Surgery,* **7:**149, 1973.

8. Cody, M. C., O'Donovan, T. P. B., and Hughes, Jr., R. W.: Idiopathic gastrointestinal bleeding and aortic stenosis. *Amer. J. Digest. Dis.* **19:**393, 1974.

9. Galloway, S. J., Casarella, W. J., and Shimkin, P. M.: Vascular malformations of the right colon as a cause of bleeding in patients with aortic stenosis. *Radiol.* **113:**11, 1974.

10. King, E. J., Baum, S., Athanasoulis, C., and Waltman, A. C.: Angiography in the diagnosis and treatment of nonvariceal bleeding in patients with portal hypertension. *Surg. Gyn. Ob.* **139:**205, 1974.

11. Athanasoulis, C. A., Brown, B., and Shapiro, J. H.: Angiography in the diagnosis and management of bleeding stress ulcers and gastritis. *Amer. J. Surg.* **125:**468, 1973.

EPILOGUE

In this book we outline a problem-oriented approach to the diagnosis and management of the patient presenting with hemorrhage from the gastrointestinal tract. Careful clinical evaluation and the application of modern diagnostic methods, such as endoscopy and angiography, permit the physician to make a precise diagnosis as to the source of the bleeding. An understanding of the physiological responses to acute blood loss should enable those caring for such patients to assure that proper cardiovascular support and resuscitation are achieved. Under these circumstances, logical and timely decisions can be made on the optimal timing of surgical intervention if it is required. To attain these goals, and thus to minimize the morbidity and mortality attending gastrointestinal hemorrhage, the physician should call on the appropriate specialists as soon as the patient arrives in the hospital. The patient's interests are best served when the specialized skills and experience of this team are fully utilized, under the guidance of one physician, who assumes the ultimate responsibility for the care of that individual patient.

INDEX